Praise for *Simply Beautiful Skin*

Simply Beautiful Skin provides clear and simple advice for attaining radiant, healthy skin. It includes valuable information for improving your nutrition and lifestyle, as well as essential instructions for selecting a minimal number of the skin care products most effective for your own age, skin and circumstances. I thoroughly enjoyed reading this book and am recommending it to all my friends and clients!

Emma Hefti
International Model, Licensed Medical Esthetician and Laser Technician at *Mint and Thyme Medical Spa*

I love Nancy's less-is-more approach to skincare! She highlights effective ingredients and simple means to get glowing skin. This skincare guide needs to be in the hands of every man and woman who wants to look and feel beautiful inside and out.

Elizabeth Ash
Licensed Esthetician, Owner of *Blessed Space Day Spa*

As a healthcare professional, I insist on effective, yet safe products. As a middle-aged woman, I expect skin care products to produce the results they promise! How often I have waded through the skin care "jungle" of overhyped promises and inflated costs. My wallet is empty, and my skin looks the same. Nancy has given us a skin care tool box to get the results we are looking for, without spending money needlessly. I highly recommend *Simply Beautiful Skin* to anyone who cares about their skin and wants to make educated and effective decisions about their product and service purchases.

Lisa K. Cauto, R.N.

The minimalist lifestyle is gaining immense popularity, while the skincare industry is exploding with new products every day. Nancy tackles both of these areas by combining her extensive skincare knowledge with reducing the noise of skincare promotional claims. How can we get the most bang for our buck while addressing our skin concerns effectively? This book provides a step-by-step guide to minimizing the number of skincare products you use, but still actively caring for your skin and its needs.

Chamagne Williams
Model, Licensed Esthetician, Owner of *Pink Daisy Beauty Bar*

Simply Beautiful Skin:

Minimize Your Skincare Routine –

Maximize the Results

Nancy Bliss

Esthetician and Holistic Skincare Advisor

Illustrated by Anastasia Goodwin

Published by BookLocker.com, Inc., St. Petersburg, Florida.

Printed on acid-free paper.

BookLocker.com, Inc.
2018

First Edition

Dedication

For Kent – you saved the day.

For Taylor and Joshua – my daily inspiration.

Disclaimer

This book details the author's personal experiences with and opinions about Skincare. The author is not a healthcare provider.

The author and publisher are providing this book and its contents on an "as is" basis and make no representations or warranties of any kind with respect to this book or its contents. The author and publisher disclaim all such representations and warranties, including for example warranties of merchantability and healthcare for a particular purpose. In addition, the author and publisher do not represent or warrant that the information accessible via this book is accurate, complete or current.

The statements made about products and services have not been evaluated by the U.S. Food and Drug Administration. They are not intended to diagnose, treat, cure, or prevent any condition or disease. Please consult with your own physician or healthcare specialist regarding the suggestions and recommendations made in this book.

Except as specifically stated in this book, neither the author or publisher, nor any authors, contributors, or other representatives will be liable for damages arising out of or in connection with the use of this book. This is a comprehensive limitation of liability that applies to all damages of any kind, including (without limitation) compensatory; direct, indirect or consequential damages; loss of data, income or profit; loss of or damage to property and claims of third parties.

You understand that this book is not intended as a substitute for consultation with a licensed healthcare practitioner, such as your physician. Before you begin any healthcare program, or change your lifestyle in any way, you will consult your physician or other licensed healthcare practitioner to ensure that you are in good health and that the examples contained in this book will not harm you.

This book provides content related to topics physical and/or mental health issues. As such, use of this book implies your acceptance of this disclaimer.

Contents

How to use this book
(and keep it simple):

If you have picked up this book, you either A: love the idea of simplifying your skincare regime and want to learn everything you can about it. Or B: you love the idea of simplifying your skincare regime but don't have a lot of free time to read a book cover to cover.

Whatever your scenario, rest assured this book was written for you. Here are three ways to use it to get the most out of the information provided and reach your individual skincare simplification goals fast.

#1: Your first choice is to read this book, in its entirety, from front to back. This option will appeal to those who love the science of skincare as it provides a solid background on skin structure, skincare ingredients, and product components; and you will learn skincare strategies for a variety of skin types and conditions.

This reading route is best if you are very interested in your skin and its care, want information on a formal nutrition program, need to know everything about an approach before trying it out, or you're interested in a thorough summary of skincare products and the industry that produces them.

For full understanding of each section, I recommend you read the book in its entirety, because many of the concepts build upon each other.

#2: Your next choice is to focus your reading on areas of the book relating to your skin type or skin condition. This option is useful if you have a basic understanding of your skin, are strapped for time, and just want to get to specific, practical suggestions.

To do this, I recommend starting with *Chapter Three: Skin Types and Conditions, and the Skincare Ingredients Best for Each*, which describes ingredients best for your skin type. You can then reference *Chapter Two: Skincare Ingredients* for more in-depth information on ingredients listed in *Chapter Three*. Next, skip over to *Chapter Six: Skin Nutrition* for nutritional guidelines specific to your skin types and condition. Lastly, choose the tear-out sheet in *Chapter Eight: Simply Beautiful Skin Regimes, Skincare Ingredients, and Nutritional Guidelines Tear-Out Sheets* applicable to your skin type or condition which you can refer to as you shop or clean out your skincare drawer (the skincare "detox").

If you need some extra motivation, you can also scan the chapters that include topics on product components, the skincare industry, spa treatments, de-stressing, and the *Simply Beautiful Skin* nutrition plan.

#3: The third option is to use this book as a workbook. This option is best for the doers, the time- starved, or those who really want to dive in after reading the book in its entirety.

- o Begin with *Chapter Eight: Simply Beautiful Skin Regimes, Skincare Ingredients, and Nutritional Guidelines Tear-Out Sheets*, and tear out the pages that apply to your skin. For example, if you have dry, sensitive, and premature aging skin, tear out the pages with those headings.
- o Then choose the skin type or condition that *most* pertains to your skin and your skincare goals and mark those pages. For example, if fine lines are really keeping you up at night, you'd choose: premature aging skin. These are the "work pages" on which you will take notes.

o Next, turn the pages you have removed from the book to the sides that list "Ingredients to look for" and "Nutritional Guidelines".

o Now turn to *Chapter Two: Skincare Ingredients* and *Chapter Three: Skin Types and Conditions, and the Skincare Ingredients Best for Each* to read about all the ingredients listed on the *Ingredients to look for* page(s) in front of you.

o Highlight on your work page the ingredients you definitely want included in your skincare   products.

o Do the same on the Nutritional Guidelines page(s), condensing suggestions specific to your needs to your work page. In our example, premature aging is the most significant concern, so highlighting and   notes were made on this page. Notes included ingredients and nutritional guidelines most applicable from the dry and sensitive pages.

o Now scan your work page and either choose "Simple A, B, or C Regime", or create your own by mixing and matching the regime components. For example, our person with premature aging skin may choose "Simple A Regime" but wants to add eye cream to his or her routine.

o Now you have a completely personalized guide to shopping for products or "detoxing" your current skincare products.

Whichever way you choose to use this book, my greatest wish is that it will serve you as a powerful and   trusted tool to help you heal your skin, simplify your life, and optimize your overall health and well-being.

In appreciation,

-*Nancy*

Introduction

It all started with bad skin and a ton of skincare products.

My battle with acne, rosacea, dermatitis, and most recently, wrinkles, led me to try every miracle-in-a- jar. My bathroom drawers and cabinets overflowed with special cleansers, creams, serums, and treatments. Desperate to solve my skin problems, I threw everything possible on my face, yet had no idea what was working and what wasn't. Yes, my skin was getting nominally better, but I was completely confused by product claims and ingredients.

Oh, and by the way, I'm an esthetician— a skincare professional who was lost in skincare products.

Then I stumbled onto a crazy and round-about way to weed through my skincare mess: the minimalist movement.

I watched a documentary called *Minimalism: A Documentary About the Important Things* because it was recommended to me, and, honestly, I was between television series on Netflix.[1] One of the most noteworthy messages of the film is that downsizing can bring peacefulness and more time to spend doing the things we love. That piqued my interest. Another idea that resonated was "the more stuff you own, the more it owns you." Was I giving up partial control of my own life by having all these things around me? Was I losing freedom to do what I wanted, when I wanted to do it? Over time, I began to reflect and ask some tough questions of myself including whether I could, possibly, live with less stuff.

One of the contributors to the film, Courtney Carver creator of *Project 333*, stood out from the others.[2] Check out her website–but in a nutshell, she challenges participants to use only 33 articles of clothing, shoes, and jewelry for 3 months. Could I do this? I read her website top to bottom and, using her tips, I cleaned my closet and clothes dressers and even parted with some items that I had saved for 20 years (I swore I was going to wear those strappy four-inch heels again one day!). I must admit that my own *Project 333* is a work in progress; I have not gotten down to 33 things yet—I'm somewhere around 80. But after that first huge closet cleaning and smaller ones since, I have found that I rarely miss what I have given away. And I do feel lighter and, dare I say, even happier.

Since my closet is a part of my bathroom, I couldn't avoid noticing the state of my bathroom cabinets and drawers, which were stuffed with cosmetics, cleansers, creams, oils, moisturizers, and serums.

Granted, I am a lotion and potion junkie, and I was looking for the best way to treat my skin conditions, but the amount I had was ridiculous. **I realized I had fallen prey to all those advertising campaigns claiming younger, healthier, clearer skin.** I would use the products for a few weeks, see no change in my skin, and then into the drawer they would be dumped. By that time, a new product would be out with even "better" claims, and soon I was on to my next miracle cure. Just lather, rinse, repeat. Perhaps you can relate?

Then a crazy thought came to me. Could I challenge myself to *minimize* my skincare products while *maximizing* my results? I decided to "rehab" my skincare routine by researching the best ingredients for specific skin concerns, so that I could discern the most effective products, and then see how much I could reduce my products while attaining better results.

I did a complete blitz of my bathroom cabinets, threw away expired products, and began investigating the ingredients in the rest. My experiment ended with reducing my daily skincare product to just the ones that benefitted my skin. (See *Chapter Three: Skin Types and Conditions, and the Skincare Ingredients Best for Each* for my personal skincare regime.)

I discovered I am not a minimalist (paring down to only the most essential items), but I want to incorporate minimalist aspects into my life, such as removing what is non-essential and focusing on what works for me. Therefore, my goal was not to create a skincare routine that is as small and short as possible, but to implement one that is effective, personalized, and uncomplicated. You will find this same philosophy throughout this book. Recommended skincare regimes, nutritional guidelines, and de- stressing techniques are first and foremost results-oriented. They are simple, but not necessarily *easy*. The case studies highlight individuals with skin types and conditions who, first and foremost, wanted to use the best products for their skin, and, secondly, wanted to reduce the quantity of skincare items. (Plus, it would be awfully boring to read about Mary who applies sunscreen in the morning and then is out the door!)

Since my own product rehab, I don't think (or overthink) anymore about my routine, and my skin has never looked better. I love the time and mind-space this has freed up. And since I'm "in the business" of skincare, if a new ingredient or product is promoted as the latest and greatest, I will consider its claims, but I've made a commitment to only try it if I can substitute it for a product I already use.

While researching products, I gained a lot of knowledge about skincare companies. I began to separate companies into three different categories:

1. The first I named "small-batch, non-corporate."
2. The second "mid-sized spa."
3. And the third was "large corporate" - the majority of skincare products fall into this group.

Large conglomerates control most of the beauty and skincare industry. In fact, seven of these companies control 182 beauty brands.[3] In the interest of full transparency, these brands also include makeup and haircare products; but the point is, many brands that *appear* independent are really controlled by large corporate companies whose main goal is to make money, not improve your skin. They do this by **charging a high price, using cheaper ingredients**, and/or **selling as many products as they can**. And, usually they employ all three tactics. In most instances, they spend more money on advertising than on research and product development.

For the sake of simplifying our understanding of the skincare industry, let's unpack the messages and tactics of most large corporate skincare lines:

Corporate Skincare Tactic #1: Charging a high price. There is nothing wrong with charging a higher price for products with quality ingredients. Higher quality products will be more effective in achieving the results you want. Also, these products can be multitaskers, so you will have fewer bottles lining your counter. Plus, you really, truly can use a lot less, making them last longer.

But, how do you know which ingredients to look for? And how do you read those unpronounceable ingredient lists? It would be great to have the knowledge to quickly scan a product list to know if you are getting your money's worth and if that product will live up to its claims. Armed with this information, you wouldn't feel pushed into buying the latest and greatest skincare product simply because they state that their blend of ingredients will work wonders. I found some of the best products have just one ingredient (and may even be found in your kitchen).

Corporate Skincare Tactic #2: Using cheaper ingredients. Large manufacturers of skincare products fill   their products with cheaper ingredients for two reasons.

First, this practice increases their profit margin (obviously).

Second, to ensure a long shelf life they must fill their products with a large quantity of typically cheap and toxic preservatives. This is especially true of drugstore and department store products. In my research, I found simple, yet highly effective products that either do not require any preservatives or, if they do, they only require the least toxin-producing ones possible.

Corporate Skincare Tactic #3: Strong-arming you into buying zillions of different products. This, in my   opinion, is the greatest scam that large, corporate companies commit. I have attended many corporate product trainings given by these companies as an esthetician, and, not all, but many skincare companies have an extensive line of products. In one training, for example, the company insisted their customers   use twelve different products in the morning and thirteen at night, plus a once-a-week exfoliation treatment. In my opinion, totally crazy!

To justify this, manufacturers will claim they need to spread out the "active ingredients" in different   products or they will become too diluted to have an effect. Really? Great moisturizers and hydrating ingredients can't be included in a product that also contains sunscreen? You can see I get a bit frustrated when these "explanations" (read: excuses) for selling more products are given.

However, keep in mind not *all* companies are like this. In today's market, there are many smaller skincare companies who do business with integrity. These are the companies I named "small batch, non-corporate." And while they still rely on profits, they have your best interests at heart.

There are also many mid-size companies that sell exclusively to spas and carry brands that focus on effectiveness in addition to their profits. Many of these skincare lines are called "cosmeceuticals." This name was created by skincare marketing to have you believe that the products are a cross between a pharmaceutical and a cosmetic, thus giving the impression that they work better than traditional skincare.

In truth, these claims are false. However, the good news is that these products may contain more active ingredients—ingredients that work to treat (such as soothe, plump, or heal) or protect your skin. Or they may contain a greater quantity of active ingredients. Usually, these skincare lines charge a pretty penny for their products, but at least you know you are getting your money's worth.

Though most spa estheticians have integrity, some earn commissions, and thus have incentive to encourage you to purchase several products at a time. If you explain your skincare goals, including your minimalist approach of using less products, in most cases you will receive honest recommendations.

However, it never hurts to have some ingredient and product knowledge under your belt, which we will cover throughout this book.

In the past, I advised my clients on what I thought was an appropriate number of products for their needs, many times bucking the suggested protocol by the manufacturer. But now, with the minimalist idea stuck in my head, my challenge became to recommend the least number of products and the easiest routine, while still delivering the same or higher level of effectiveness.

My research, subsequent changes in my personal skincare regime, and my work with clients, were the motivation behind this book. I want to give you just enough information to make the best, yet simplest, choices for your skincare regime.

Regarding your skincare, this book will help you:

- o Reduce the number of skincare products you use;
- o Choose the most effective skincare products based on the knowledge of what ingredients work   best for your skin type or condition;
- o Detect whether a product contains a sufficient amount of active ingredients and minimal   amount of fillers, preservatives, colors, and fragrances;
- o Choose foods that support healthy, vibrant skin, and gain knowledge of foods that address   particular skin conditions;
- o Discern if a spa treatment should be in your skincare regime;
- o Empower you to be able to weed through (or ignore) those ubiquitous skincare ads,
- o Save time and energy for more worthwhile endeavors;
- o And most importantly, feel amazing after your own skincare rehab with radiant, healthy skin.

What you will learn:

- o In this book, we will start with the basics of skin anatomy.
- o Then, we will dive into understanding key ingredients (including ingredients for specific skin   conditions).
- o Next, typical products are defined with suggestions of simple non-commercial substitutions; this   is followed by a discussion of spa/facial treatments and why they may make your daily skincare   routine easier.
- o Then, we will cover nutrition and food choice information, because so much of our skin health is   determined internally.
- o Next, you will learn a simple de-stressing technique to help stave off the signs of skin stress,   including breakouts, premature aging, and more.

- o And lastly, we will put it all together with nifty tear-out sample skincare routines based on your skin type or condition.

My hope in publishing this book is that you will find information to make confident decisions about the type and number of skincare products you really need. My goal is for you to choose products that are the most effective, so that you can reduce the number of products you use.

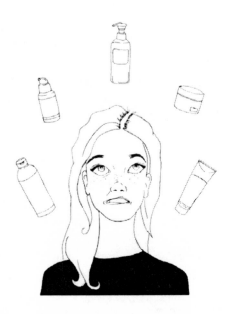

How might this look for you? Maybe you will get down to using only one product in the morning and at night. Perhaps you will be able to pare down your products so that you can see to the bottom of your bathroom drawers. And, maybe because you are armed with knowledge, you will be able to wave off most or all the 25 products the salesperson at the beauty counter encourages you to buy.

My ultimate wish is that you find this philosophy to be one facet of a life of reduced stress, saving time, and accomplishing more with less, while attaining beautiful, glowing skin!

Chapter One: Skin Basics 101

You probably want to skip over this chapter and get to the "good" stuff, right?

While it may be tempting to skip, having a working knowledge of your skin's biology will help you understand the ingredients in future chapters and choose the best product for your skin concerns and goals. I promise to keep it simple—just like the philosophy of this book.

The skin is our largest organ and is involved in Vitamin D synthesis, protection from environmental assaults, body temperature regulation, water retention in the body, immune system function, and toxin removal from the body. It acts as a barrier to the outside world and is highly interconnected with our other organs and systems.

Its health can be affected extrinsically (from the environment) and intrinsically (from internal functions). Damaging external factors include UV rays, bacteria, wind, air pollution, and skincare products. It is also   important to know that approximately 70 percent of what is placed on the skin will be absorbed into our bloodstreams.

This is why many are concerned about toxins in skincare. If you wouldn't eat it, why put it on your skin?

The lesser known component of skin health is intrinsic health. This includes diet, exercise, and physical activity. Though it is not commonplace to consider the implications of intrinsic health and skincare, more and more studies are finding that what we eat has an impact on our skin.

One study found that the formation of wrinkles was influenced by foods in the diet.[4] Participants who ate beans, vegetables, and olive oil in their diet had the lowest level of visible skin aging, and those who ate a diet high in meat, dairy, and butter had the highest. This is just one example of many studies demonstrating a strong correlation between diet and skin health. More recently, studies suggest a link between exercising and improving skin regeneration.[5]

In addition, smoking is an internal toxin that has been found to greatly affect the health of skin. Smoking reduces oxygen and blood flow to the skin, leaving it dry and discolored. It also depletes your skin of many nutrients including vitamin C that helps protect against premature aging and sun damage.[6]

But, before we dive into what is best to put on your skin and in your body to improve your skin health, let's look at skin itself.

There are three main layers of your skin: the epidermis, the dermis, and the hypodermis (subcutaneous fat layer).

LAYERS OF YOUR SKIN

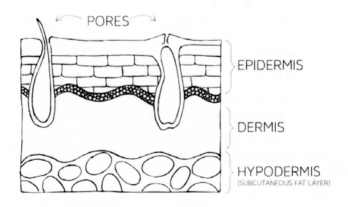

PORES

EPIDERMIS

DERMIS

HYPODERMIS
(SUBCUTANEOUS FAT LAYER)

The Epidermis

The epidermis is the outermost layer, and it is the layer most affected by what we do, or don't do, to our skin. It contains four different types of cells:

- **Keratinocytes** produce keratin, which is a protein that protects the body against bacteria, heat, and harmful chemicals.
- **Merkel cells** are responsible for the sensation of touch.
- **Langerhans cells**, a part of the immune system, produce antibodies that fight infection.
- **And Melanocytes** produce the melanin that is responsible for the color of the skin and any darker areas on the skin such as freckles, sun spots, or melasma (a darkened area or areas on the face caused by hormonal changes, especially during pregnancy). Any skin condition that includes dark areas, but especially sun damage in the form of uneven skin tone, is also called hyperpigmentation.

The epidermis sloughs off and regenerates every month or so, although this process slows with age. Located at the deepest level of the epidermis, cells (named basal cells) multiply and divide, pushing the older cells up to the surface until they are shed from the skin. The jury is still out, but there are products that claim to speed up this process by stimulating the basal cells.

An important component of the epidermis is the acid mantle. The acid mantle is made up of oils produced by the body called sebum, salts, and the top layer of dead skin cells. This acid mantle acts as a barrier to protect against outside elements. This is called its "barrier function".

Any means of exfoliation—such as manual (scrubs or machines), chemical (retinoids and peels), or laser— will remove the top layer of dead cells, leaving a fresher, glowing complexion. However, it is important not to harm the acid mantle by over-exfoliating or by using overly harsh products, because this can cause skin conditions such as rosacea; or, if you have oily skin, it will encourage your cells to produce more oil. Plus, sebum is responsible for keeping skin soft and killing bacteria, so continually stripping the acid mantle can lead to dry, problematic skin.

The acid mantle also protects against too much transepidermal water loss, or TEWL. TEWL is a normal function of the body where water from inside the body passes through the skin and is evaporated.

However, if this action is allowed to go into overdrive by a compromised barrier, it will lead to dehydration, inflammation and, possibly, an adverse skin condition.

Another significant aspect of the epidermis is an ecosystem called the microbiome, or skin flora. This system of healthy bacteria is responsible for eliminating toxins expelled through sweat. One reason we experience body odor after sweating comes from the bacteria consuming those toxins.

In addition, healthy bacteria keep harmful bacteria in check. Acne, for example, is caused by harmful bacteria named *Propionibacterium acne (P. acnes)*, which means we can reduce breakouts by keeping the skin microbiome healthy. Skin flora also protects against invasions of harmful organisms while helping educate your immune system's T cells to attack pathogens.[7]

It's amazing all this is happening in and on our skin.

Many more studies are being done to expand our knowledge of the skin microbiome, but what we know now is that a healthy diet that includes probiotic foods can help strengthen this system.

However, it is important to know that off-the-shelf skincare products that claim to include probiotics that will help your skin are pulling your leg. Probiotics cannot exist with preservatives, and any off-the- shelf products that include water (which are most) require preservatives. If you want to give your skin a *real* probiotic treatment, you will need to "Do-It-Yourself." (See *Chapter Four: Skincare Products* for a DIY Probiotic Skin Balancing Mask recipe or apply plain yogurt that includes probiotic strains of bacteria as a mask.)

The Dermis

The dermis is located below the epidermis and is made up mainly of the proteins collagen and elastin. Collagen gives skin strength, volume, and resilience. Elastin makes it flexible. Both of these components play a huge role in supporting skin's youthful appearance. Unfortunately, as we age, production slows down and both proteins become stiffer and more brittle, leading to sagging and wrinkles. In addition, both extrinsic and intrinsic factors can affect the production and health of collagen and elastin. Sun damage and exposure to other free radicals are major contributors to the breakdown of these proteins, as are hormonal changes, poor diet, inflammation, and stress.

Despite the many skincare products making outlandish claims about so-called "anti-aging ingredients," it is important to know that **it has not been definitively proven that any ingredient can sink into the dermis to rev up collagen and elastin production**. However, throughout this book you will read claims from studies that have shown various ingredients increasing collagen and elastin production. How this happens is not completely known. One reason could be that collagen and elastin regeneration is indirectly stimulated by the reaction of the skin to specific skincare products. For example, exfoliators accelerate cell turnover and this action may boost creation of these skin-building blocks.

What is accepted is that SPF in sunscreen protects against harmful sun rays, antioxidants (both in products and in the diet) guard against free radicals, and a healthy diet will help balance hormones and reduce, or even alleviate, many types of inflammation, which can lead to a reduction in collagen and elastin production.

The Hypodermis

The deepest layer of the skin is the hypodermis, or subcutaneous fat layer, which, as the name suggests, is a layer of fat. This cushion, along with water, plumps the skin, creating a healthy, youthful appearance.

The importance of our skin goes way beyond just looks. This essential organ is our body's greatest   protector. Therefore, as we take care of our body and mind with nourishing food, exercise, and de- stressing activities, we are more than half-way to accomplishing our skin goals. Sure, we still need to   take care of our skin from the outside, but the practice of working on our skin from the inside out greatly simplifies our need for multiple skincare products.

Chapter Two: Skincare Ingredients

As an independent esthetician, I am lucky to have worked with many clients to try out different treatments using various skincare products and product lines. My work has allowed me to tweak my treatments based on months and years of results. I modified my work regularly by adding ancient therapies and tonics, like Ayurvedic lymph massage and essential oils. This freedom gave me the opportunity to search out and apply best practices with the most effective ingredients.

What follows is information on ingredients found in many skincare products I have researched and used.

You may think I've abandoned the "simple" theme of this book based on the extensiveness of this inventory; however, having a bit of background information on ingredients will help you to make better product choices for life. Or, if you prefer, you can use this chapter as a reference for future shopping trips.

This list is not exhaustive; new ingredients are being touted in products all the time. Also, there are thousands of additional ingredients such as emulsifiers, polymers, and fillers. For a complete list check out the "bible of skincare ingredients", *Milady Skincare and Cosmetic Ingredients Dictionary*, in which over 2,300 ingredients are defined. Thrilling reading if you are a cosmetic ingredient nerd like me!

In keeping with our theme of simplicity and results, included in this chapter are "active" ingredients (ingredients that are beneficial to your skin rather than ingredients that make a product cohesive or shelf-stable) that have been proven to be effective, have been used in many skincare lines, and/or are typically included in specific type products.

As I am a holistic esthetician, my expertise (and admitted bias) is in more natural and less toxin-producing ingredients that actually work. Therefore, the information below will reflect this; however, my focus will be on the *effectiveness* of the ingredient. I have found most natural ingredients to be just as effective, or *more* effective, than manufactured ingredients.

However, in the interest of effectiveness and results, I have included some controversial ingredients sometimes deemed "toxic." I include them because they can be highly advantageous in solving a nagging or even severe skin condition, and I only recommend these types of ingredients when a natural ingredient does not address the issue as effectively.

I believe the true concept of holistic treatment is to consider ALL treatment options to discern the best skincare regime for you. However, it is important to keep in mind that approximately 70 percent of what is put on the skin goes directly into the bloodstream. Therefore, it is best to weigh the benefits of controversial ingredients with the suggested toxicity.

I also use the term "natural" in a general sense, meaning made in nature or chemically derived from elements found in nature. Use of the "natural" label by mass manufacturers is just a maneuver to make us *think* the product is better for our skin and health in general. True natural products needn't use that tactic.

Many terms used in the marketing of products (especially mass-produced) don't really mean all that much. Organic ingredients are different as they must be certified by the government to legally use the term "organic." But unless it is important for you to fully support organic farming, I wouldn't put much concern into that label. Many smaller manufacturers include ingredients grown organically, yet they cannot afford the certification. And, many times it is better to buy from these small-batch, non- corporate businesses because they tend to be more transparent in their labeling and advertising.

Because of my more-natural approach, the fact that natural ingredients in many instances work better than the man-made version, and that most people I have worked with would rather use natural products, you will see the word "botanical" quite a bit in this section. Botanicals are ingredients derived from plants, commonly herbs, roots, flowers, fruits, leaves, or seeds. When you are reading a skincare product label, if you see the word "extract" after the ingredient, it is a botanical, meaning it is extracted from the plant.

Before we dig into specific ingredients, I want to talk about two words used in skincare that can sound scary or intimidating: acids and chemicals. In the skincare world, these terms are sometimes used interchangeably, such as chemical peels and acid peels. Acids are chemicals. Chemicals can come from nature or be man-made. They are simply a substance with a molecule structure that is either produced by a process or used in a process. For example, fruit acids are chemicals. When choosing an ingredient that is a chemical (in that it will cause a chemical reaction such as exfoliation), it is best to choose a naturally-occurring one if you use it on a regular basis (such as once a week or more), because your body recognizes chemicals from nature easier than man-made chemicals. Because of this, many believe any synthetic chemical is a toxin.

Stronger peels offered in spas or dermatologists' offices typically include man-made acids or a blend, including synthetic acids. These peels are usually applied once a month or once a year, so you will need to decide whether the benefits outweigh the possible toxicity.

When the word "acid" is mentioned, an image of battery acid burning through metal may come to mind. In skincare, you might think of a solution that burns skin down to the dermis. And while there are skincare acids that can do this (found in dermatologists' offices), most acids are much gentler, especially acids derived from plants or fruit. An acid is an agent that releases hydrogen ions when added to water and has a pH of less than 7. In skincare terms, acids cause a variety of actions, such as exfoliation, hydration, brightening, and protection against environmental damage. If an ingredient ends with the word "acid," it doesn't necessarily mean that it will peel the skin. There is an acid for just about any skin issue, including dry skin, fine lines, and acne.

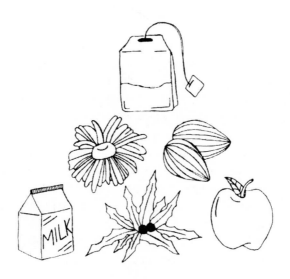

Types of Ingredients

Exfoliators

I love, love, LOVE exfoliators! Now that I've gotten that out of my system, let me explain.

Remember the cell regeneration process explained in Chapter One: Skin Basics 101? Well, exfoliation removes that top layer of dead skin cells on the epidermis.

Your skin regenerates on its own, so applying chemicals is not necessary, but it does have many benefits including:

o   Exfoliating allows fresher, brighter cells to shine on the top layer of your skin. With the uppermost dead skin cells removed, serums and treatment products will be more effective since they will be able to penetrate better.
o   It aids in lessening skin pigmentation over time by breaking up the darker skin cells and allowing them to fade.
o   Acne and pimples heal more quickly with regular chemical exfoliation.

In addition, it signals our skin to push more cells to the surface (since the top microscopic layer was removed), so the regeneration process is revved up. Since this process slows as we age, we are tricking our skin into acting younger. Some exfoliators absorb deeper into the skin and claim to repair the layers where collagen and elastin reside, leading to smoother, more resilient skin. By activating the collagen and elastin, the deeper layers of the skin thicken, causing increased skin firmness. In other words: these babies can really transform the skin! You can opt for daily exfoliators (such as a nightly retinol treatment or a brightening serum), a weekly product (such as an alpha and beta hydroxy acid mask), or a monthly facial from a spa, from a beauty school, or done at home.

NOTE: more is not necessarily better in the case of exfoliators, as you do not want to disrupt the acid mantle and skin flora by overusing them. **Cut back on or temporarily eliminate exfoliation if your skin becomes sensitive, red, or if the problems you are trying to correct get worse.** There are exfoliating ingredients that are beneficial for most skin types and conditions, including rosacea. But even these milder, therapeutic exfoliation ingredients can be over used. In addition, **always use a sunscreen when using exfoliators on a regular basis.** The strength of over-the-counter products containing chemical exfoliators can range between 0.5 or ½ percent to 10 percent, while professional concentrations can contain 20 to 70 percent. At home, it is best to start with the lowest concentration and slowly increase the percentage of concentration as you replace depleted products, if you desire more exfoliation.

Alpha Hydroxy Acids (AHAs)): Natural Acids Found in Foods

Glycolic Acid is found in sugar cane. It is a wonderful exfoliator, especially for premature aging skin. Since it is a smaller molecule than other AHAs, caution should be taken when beginning use as it will penetrate more layers faster, which could lead to burning. It is this characteristic that allows it to sink deeper into the skin, increasing its benefits as an exfoliator. If you have darker skin, glycolic acid has been shown to cause more irritation than other acids.

Mandelic Acid is found in bitter almonds. This is a more versatile, gentler acid appropriate for all skin shades. It has been shown to help fine lines, acne, and hyperpigmentation (sun or dark spots), while also supporting the skin through its strengthening and rejuvenating characteristics. It is both anti- inflammatory and antibacterial, making it ideal for very sensitive or inflamed skin (in smaller doses).

Malic Acid is commonly found in apples. This acid will brighten the skin as an exfoliator and works as a hydrator by pulling moisture to the skin. It also has better buffering capabilities, which means you can use more of it without upsetting the acid mantle pH balance.

Lactic Acid is found in milk. This is the gentlest AHA and is fantastic for premature aging and dry skin because it conditions and hydrates as it exfoliates. Milk baths have been used for centuries to smooth and soften the skin—all due to the lactic acid. Do not use it if you have acne or blemish-prone skin.

Azelaic Acid is found in whole grains and is one of the best-kept secrets for rosacea, acne, hyperpigmentation, or all the above. Like salicylic acid, it works as an anti-inflammatory, yet is much gentler, making it highly effective for both the pustules and redness of rosacea.

For acne, it is antibacterial and controls sebum production (like salicylic acid), while aiding in regulating cell production, so they don't build up and clog the pores.

For hyperpigmentation, it has been shown to target pigment-producing cells while leaving normal ones alone, which makes it excellent for all skin tones. Therefore, you can treat your acne while also helping fade the dark spots blemishes leave behind.

One drawback to azelaic acid is that a high level of the acid is needed to see marked results; therefore, professional treatments or a prescription medication is suggested. For over the counter products, look for its derivative, **azeloyl glycine**, which requires less dosage.

There are other AHAs, such as tartaric acid (from grapes) and citric acid (from citrus fruits), but they are less common in skincare products.

Beta Hydroxy Acids (BHAs)

BHAs are chemically similar to AHAs, yet they are oil-soluble rather than water-soluble. This oil solubility allows them to penetrate deeper into the pores of the skin, especially oily skin. The only BHA used in skincare is **Salicylic Acid,** which can be also listed as **Willow Bark**. Many times, it is simply listed on the label as **BHA**. It is the best treatment for acne since it dissolves impactions in the pores that make up blemishes and blackheads. It also reduces sebum (oil) secretion, which is important because oil will clog pores and attract the acne-causing bacteria, *P. acnes*. In addition, its anti-inflammatory properties will calm irritated, red skin, making it ideal for those with rosacea and sensitive skin. Be sure to use a lower concentration at first. Start with 2 percent and slowly move up to no more than 15 percent. Do not use if you have very dry skin or if you are pregnant.

Enzymes

Enzymes exfoliate by digesting keratin, the dead skin cells that make up the top layers of the epidermis, leading to smoother skin. Common enzymes come from fruit including **papaya (papain), pumpkin (*Cucurbita pepo*), pineapple (bromelain), and blueberry enzymes**. Papaya enzyme is also an anti- inflammatory, making it excellent for people with sensitive skin or rosacea. Pumpkin and pineapple are the strongest enzymes, with pineapple containing the added benefit of vitamin C, an antioxidant. In fact, all these fruit enzymes include phytochemicals that also act as antioxidants.

Retinol

Most people have heard of the prescription medication Retin-A® (medically known as tretinoin), a topical retinoic acid that may be named **retinyl palmitate** on the ingredient list. It is a stable form of vitamin A shown to prevent wrinkles and soften existing wrinkles. As an aggressive exfoliator, it is also frequently prescribed for acne. However, users complain it has an extremely drying effect and can cause redness, itching, burning, and visible peeling. Chemists and skin experts have found these negative effects occur because of tretinoin's large molecules, which cannot penetrate the skin easily, resulting in irritation of the top layers of skin. This irritation also happens because tretinoin is a highly concentrated retinoic acid (a form of vitamin A). Retinol is different in that it is made up of smaller molecules, less concentrated, and converts to retinoic acid in the skin, making it gentler even if it takes longer to see results.

Retinol is a game-changing ingredient, and one of my favorites, because of its proven effectiveness in promoting a clear complexion, smoothing uneven skin texture, increasing cell turnover which may boost collagen production, fading hyperpigmentation, and reducing fine lines and wrinkles. It is fantastic for skin that is aging prematurely and for delaying the signs of aging for as long as possible.

Because retinol can be drying, you must build up your skin's tolerance for it. Start with 0.5 or ½ percent and move up in concentration as your skin allows. The highest concentration you can buy over the counter is 2 ½ or 2.5 percent. It is also wonderful for blemish-prone skin. Just be careful to choose the right retinol product–one that contains retinol plus salicylic acid and that is made for acneic skin.

Do not use retinol products if you are pregnant, and be aware that it breaks down rapidly when exposed to sunlight, so use only at night and wear sunscreen during the day.

Antioxidants

Whether an antioxidant is used on the skin or eaten as part of your diet, it does the same work; it   prevents or slows down oxidation caused by the effects of free radicals.

To understand better, let's do a short chemistry lesson. Free radicals are formed when an oxygen atom   loses an electron. The electron, now terribly unstable, steals an electron from another substance so that   it can become stable again. However, this is damaging to the cell and its functions, including collagen   cells and their production. This process can also spark a chain reaction where millions (or more) of free   radicals are formed within seconds.

Countless aspects of our modern society cause free radicals, including:

o   pesticides,
o   air pollution,
o   cigarette smoke,
o   poor food choices,
o   and, the worst culprit, UV rays from the sun.

Your skin has natural protections against free radical damage, yet the problem occurs when the quantity   of free radicals exceeds what your body can handle. Plus, this ability to fight off free radicals diminishes   with age. **The number one culprit of skin aging is free radical activity.**[8]

Enter antioxidants—your skin's superhero! Vitamin C is the most common antioxidant skincare   ingredient by far, but there are many more, including vitamin E, zeaxanthin, astaxanthin, resveratrol,   and green tea extract. Apply antioxidants in the morning before you apply sunscreen to increase sun   protection.

Vitamin C comes in many forms, but the most common are **Ascorbic Acid, Ascorbyl Palmate, Ascorbyl   Palmitate** and **Magnesium Ascorbyl Phosphate (MAP).** While ascorbic acid is known to be the gold-   standard, studies have shown that magnesium ascorbyl phosphate works just as well and is gentler on   the skin (magnesium ascorbyl phosphate converts to ascorbic acid once it penetrates the skin). Vitamin C   is a tried-and-true protector of UV ray oxidation and, in some studies, one application's protection can   last three days (even after washing the face).[9] Along with its protective abilities, vitamin C is also a   wonderful skin brightener, can help even out skin tone, and potentially aids in increasing the production   of collagen. N

Vitamin E, also listed as a form of **tocopherol,** is the free radical fighting partner of vitamin C. They are   the Batman and Robin of antioxidants! Vitamin C repairs vitamin E after it attacks a free radical so that it can go on fighting those free radical criminals. In addition, vitamin E helps protect against cell damage from inflammation when applied before sun exposure. It also works as a moisturizer as well as a hydrator, and has been shown to reduce skin pigmentation and counteract the decrease in oil production as we age. Note that pure Vitamin E oil can be very sticky and thick.

Zeaxanthin and **Astaxanthin** are fairly new to the antioxidant skincare party. Both are carotenoids— pigments that give plants their color. Zeaxanthin is found in leafy green vegetables, yellow and orange peppers, and eggs. Astaxanthin is similar to beta-carotene and is found in marine animals, such as salmon and shrimp. Both are purported to be more beneficial than vitamin C in free radical protection. Astaxanthin, especially, proved to be much more effective as an antioxidant than either vitamin C or E.[10] If skin studies conclude the same as the nutrition studies, we will be seeing both ingredients more in skincare products.

Another antioxidant studied first in the diet was **Resveratrol,** found in red grape skins. Suddenly we had an excuse to drink a glass of red wine each night! (It is also found in dark chocolate, if that helps you feel better about that Ghirardelli square for dessert).

More recently, studies have shown resveratrol applied to the skin has antioxidant abilities 58 percent   more efficient than vitamin C.[11] And as a bonus, it is reported to increase collagen content in the skin by stimulating fibroblasts, the cells that create collagen.[12]

Green Tea Extract also works double duty by combating oxidation and inflammation in the skin. This is a   great antioxidant for sensitive skin or rosacea. Green tea contains EGCg (epigallocatechin gallate), a plant compound with antioxidant properties, which protects from UV rays and other free radicals, and   has been shown to help sustain the life of fibroblasts.[13] Additionally, extracts of **White Tea**, **Red Tea**, **Black Tea,** and **Rooibos Tea** are also excellent antioxidants.

There are a host of other substances used as antioxidants in skincare, including, but not limited to, **Grapeseed** *(Vitia vinifera)*, **Coffee Berry**, and **Alpha Lipoic Acid** (*Thioctic acid*). Many of these are used in combination with the other antioxidants described here for more beneficial synergistic effects.

Hydrators

Hydrators, also called humectants, pull water from the air and bind it to your skin. Though there are many hydrating ingredients, the list below only includes natural or chemically-derived substances that the skin recognizes, which enables them to perform more effectively.

Hyaluronic Acid is currently the hottest hydrator found in skincare products, because it occurs naturally throughout our bodies, including in the dermis, eyes, and joints. In the dermis, it regulates water content, elasticity, and the distribution of nutrients. A common misconception about Hyaluronic Acid is that if it is applied to the skin, it will penetrate all the way to the dermis and effectively join the body's concentration of this substance. Unfortunately, the topically-applied hyaluronic acid is too large of a molecule to absorb that deeply.

But, that does not mean it is ineffective in skincare—quite the opposite—it is *the premier hydrator*, an anti-aging powerhouse, and good for all skin types. As a hydrator, it holds an amazing 1,000 times its weight in water, yet when applied it won't disrupt acid mantle balance. And for bonus points, it works as an antioxidant while making the skin smoother, resulting in less noticeable wrinkles and lines.

Note: you may see **Sodium Hyaluronate** on a product's ingredient list. This is a salt derived from hyaluronic acid and has all the same benefits, and it is more easily absorbed.

Glycerin is, by far, the most common hydrating ingredient in skincare products. It has been studied   extensively and has been found to be a good hydrating agent. And as a byproduct of soap making, it is   also very pure.

Honey, like many ingredients straight from nature, has many beneficial qualities, including hydrating the   skin. It is also an antioxidant and is loaded with enzymes which gently exfoliate the skin. Honey also is   excellent for balancing the skin's microbiome or flora. For convenient application, try making your own   facial mask to use at night, or choose a product that contains honey.

Emollients

Emollients act as an occlusive—a substance that forms a barrier on the skin so that moisture does not   evaporate. Moisturizers are mixtures of ingredients that must contain an emollient such as:

- o   Plant oils
- o   Animal oils, such as emu, mink, or lanolin
- o   Petroleum-based oils, such as mineral oil or enzymes
- o   Esters, which are formed from a chemical reaction of combining fatty alcohols and an acid while   removing water. Esters are components of oils, butters, and waxes and are completely safe.
- o   Ceramides are fats and come from plants, such as wheat germ, or can be made synthetically. Ceramides are effective and safe.
- o   Cholesterol, which is a fat-like substance found in plant and animal cells. It is very safe.
- o   Butters
- o   Waxes
- o   Aloe vera gel or extract

The best oils for the skin are derived from vegetables, plants, seeds, and nuts, and there is an oil for   every skin type. Emu oil (from the emu bird) is included below because it has such beneficial properties. Butters, like oils, are fats; however, they are consistently solid. Because they are so emollient, most   butters are included in body care products rather than facial care. One exception is shea butter; it is used in both facial and body skincare. Waxes are harder, but less greasy than oils and butters. They are   usually part of a blend of ingredients in a moisturizer since most are too hard to use on their own.

Waxes are more resistant to oxidation than oils or butters, so they have a longer shelf life. And aloe vera   gel or extract is in a class all its own.

Some emollients are ingredients in skincare products or are stand-alone products, such as facial oils.

Regarding facial oil, it is imperative to look for quality to ensure that all the beneficial properties are   intact. Some key words or phrases to look for are:

- o   "USDA Certified Organic" (although, as noted earlier, small companies may not be able to afford   this certification)
- o   "Cold-pressed"
- o   "Unrefined"

If you don't find these descriptions on the label, make sure you are buying from a reputable company. Sometimes the largest brands in health food stores are not the best, therefore I recommend smaller companies for their superior products. If you are in doubt of how the company processes its emollients,   and they are not transparent on their website, call them up. I have, and I let them convince me that they   produce a worthy product. If they are stumped when you ask about their practices, or they transfer you   into oblivion, then you may want to pass.

Another point to consider: you usually get what you pay for with all base skincare ingredients. This   doesn't mean you need to purchase the most expensive brand; however, if the product is super cheap, it may contain additives or be adulterated in some way, negating its value.

When it comes to oils, don't be put off if an oil is darker in color or has a distinct smell—unless it smells "bad" or rancid. Very light-colored, translucent oils are usually refined and, unfortunately, nutrient value   is lost with this process. Oils should be kept in a dark-colored glass bottle in a fairly cool environment.

You can preserve their freshness and shelf-life by storing in the refrigerator, but they may solidify; this   doesn't hurt the oil, and you can simply take it out of the refrigerator at least an hour before use. If kept   at room temperature, use them up within a year, except where noted below.

Olive Oil *(Olea europaea oil)* is a medium-weight oil and contains antioxidants, such as vitamin E,   essential fatty acids, and squalane. It is very emollient and, therefore, great for dry skin. When choosing an olive oil, look for extra-virgin and cold-pressed. This ensures it contains the greatest amount of   antioxidants and other bio-nutrients.

Squalane, as mentioned above, is found in olive oil. It also occurs naturally in the body and can be   derived from sharks' livers or olives (for ethical reasons, please make sure the squalane you choose is produced from olives). Squalane's chemical makeup is identical to your body's own oil (sebum), is non- greasy feeling, *and* replenishes your skin's acid mantel, making it a highly beneficial ingredient in moisturizers. It also has a lovely silky texture.

Note: don't mistake *squalane* with *squalene*. Squalene oxidizes more quickly.

Hazelnut Oil *(Corylus avellane)* is a gentle, moisturizing nut oil that also helps regulate sebum production. It is best for oily, normal, or combination skin, is light and fast-absorbing, and contains vitamin E and other antioxidants.

Avocado Oil *(Persea gratissima oil)* is a heavier oil, best for deep moisturizing. It is also very gentle and, because it penetrates deeper than many other oils, makes it ideal for sensitive, dry, or flaky skin. If your skin runs hot or red, this oil has a cooling effect. It also contains a natural sunscreen (but may be too heavy to wear during the day) and vitamins A, D, and E, as well as sterolins, which are natural steroids that may boost collagen and treat age spots.

Simple Beauty Tip: For a quick, hydrating mask, try rubbing mashed avocado on your face.

Hemp Seed Oil *(Cannabis sativa oil)* comes from the cannabis plant, but does not contain THC, the active ingredient in marijuana. If this makes you uncomfortable, keep in mind that many items are made from hemp, including paper, protein powder, and cloth. It is a versatile, sustainable plant that has been cultivated for thousands of years. It contains antioxidants, essential fatty acids, and vitamins A, D, and E. It is also anti-inflammatory, making it good for decreasing redness and irritation in sensitive and acne- prone skin.

Rice Bran Oil *(Oryza sativa bran oil)* is the oil extracted from the germ and inner husks of rice. It is known for its soothing enzymes and antioxidant properties and contains vitamins A, B2, B12, and E. This oil is very popular with Japanese men and women, who have used it for ages for skin conditioning.

Grapeseed Oil *(Vitis vinifera oil)* is fantastic for oily skin as it helps regulate the production of sebum. It is a light oil that is absorbed quickly into the skin and is also astringent, meaning it can constrict the pores.

Borage Seed Oil (*Borago officinalis oil*) is very calming, healing, and emollient, making it good for dry, damaged, and sensitive skin. It contains high amounts of omega-6 fatty acids and has the most gamma linolenic acid (GLA) of any seed oil—GLA is beneficial for these skin types.

Neem Seed Oil (*Azadirachta indica oil*), which comes from a seed from a tree native to India, has been a staple skincare oil in the Ayurveda community for centuries. It fights all infections as it is antibacterial, antifungal, and antiviral. Because of this, and the fact that it is anti-inflammatory, this oil is best for acne-prone skin. It is well absorbed, but, beware, it has a very strong scent.

Sea Buckthorn Seed Oil (*Hippophae rhamnoides oil*) is derived from the berry seeds of a shrub native to Asia. This oil has an almost cult following because of its many beneficial properties. It is rich in vitamin E, and contains vitamins A and C. It is highly regenerating, healing, anti-inflammatory, and antibacterial. It also contains a natural sunscreen. It absorbs quickly into the skin and is beneficial for all skin types, except very oily or blemish-prone skin.

Argan Oil (*Argania spinosa oil*) is obtained from the nut of the argan tree grown only in Morocco. This oil definitely lives up to the hype. It is best for dry and wrinkle-prone skin. Like pure vitamin E oil, it has been shown to help the appearance of stretch marks and is best known for its skin-firming capabilities and for making the skin suppler. This oil has a shelf life of about two years.

Rosehip Seed Oil (*Rosa moschata seed oil*) is a personal favorite for many skin types, especially skin that is aging prematurely. This multitasking oil is a natural source of retinoic acid (vitamin A), acts as a hydrator and a moisturizer, has natural sunscreen capabilities, and is loaded with nutrients and essential fatty acids.

One caveat: only use in concentrations of 20 percent or less, as it may cause redness and irritation in higher concentrations.

Therefore, if you are making your own skincare formulations, mix with other oils such as marula, argan, avocado, jojoba, or cranberry seed oil.

Marula Oil (*Sclerocarya birrea oil*) is another multitasking oil boasting a high level of antioxidants (including vitamins C and E), abundant essential fatty acids, and is both hydrating and antibacterial, making it good for blemish-prone skin. It also has a smaller molecular make-up, allowing it to penetrate more layers of skin and absorb quicker than some other oils. This is an excellent oil for all skin types.

Coconut Oil (*Cocos nucifera oil*) has become the new darling of nutrition and skincare. It is highly emollient and naturally changes consistency with temperature changes. It contains a high amount of vitamin E and other beneficial nutrients; however, it is comedogenic, meaning it clogs pores. This may be due to its tendency to be poorly absorbed by the skin. Use only if you have extremely dry skin, and do not use on acne-prone skin. This oil has a shelf life of about two years.

Cranberry Seed Oil (*Vaccinium macrocarpon oil*) contains two forms of vitamin E: tocopherols and tocotrienols. This rare trait makes it a good antioxidant oil. It is also rich in essential fatty acids, especially omega-3. This oil has a shelf life of about two years.

Evening Primrose Oil (*Oenothera biennis oil*) is a light, easily-absorbed oil great for sensitive skin. If you suffer from psoriasis, eczema, or dermatitis, this is the oil for you. It helps to heal (some claim cure) these conditions by reducing skin redness and alleviating itchiness. Additionally, it contains essential fatty acids and helps to boost blood circulation. This is a fragile oil that requires refrigeration.

Calendula Oil (*Calendula officinalis oil*) is extracted from the calendula or marigold blossom. It is known for its repairing, wound-healing, soothing, antibacterial, and anti-inflammatory properties, making it a wonderful oil for oily, acne-prone, and sensitive skin. It is gentle, cooling, and stimulates collagen at wound sites, minimizing scarring.

Emu Oil (*Dromaius novae hollandiae oil*) is a wildly popular oil that comes from the emu bird. This super- beneficial oil is made up of 70 percent essential fatty acids and has a balanced amount of omega-9, 6, and 3. It is anti-inflammatory, contains the antioxidant vitamin E and is rich in vitamin A. This oil is similar to the sebum produced by the skin, so it absorbs quickly without a greasy feel. It is especially good for mature skin, as advocates claim that it thickens the skin while making it plumper and healthier. Emu oil is also good to help treat psoriasis and eczema.

Note that this oil may smell slightly "gamey," and you should look for oil that comes from birds that are humanely raised and not given hormones or medicines. As it is a delicate oil, it should be kept refrigerated.

Shea Butter (*Butyrospermum parkii*) is obtained from shea tree nuts found in West Africa. It is a versatile cream that can treat skin allergies, sunburn, insect bites, and minor wounds. The oil in shea butter mimics the sebum produced by the skin, which, along with its naturally-occurring vitamins A and E, makes it a great facial moisturizer. It is best for dry and/or irritated skin.

Jojoba Oil (*Simmondsia chinensis*) is another one of my favorites, despite that it isn't even an oil at all. It is a liquid wax that has been held in high regard by Native Americans for its cosmetic and healing properties. Look for jojoba oil that is golden in color and has a nutty aroma, which indicates it is non- refined and has retained all of its beneficial properties. It is almost a perfect match, structurally and chemically, to sebum, allowing it to penetrate better without leaving a greasy feel. It is antibacterial, contains antioxidants, and has a high level of vitamin E. It is a fantastic moisturizer for all skin types, including acne, because it tricks your skin into thinking it has produced enough sebum. In addition, it has a five-year shelf life—much longer than other facial oils.

Aloe Extract or **Aloe Vera Gel** (*Aloe barbadensis*) is a super cooling botanical that is antibiotic, hydrating, moisturizing, and acts as a wound healer. It interferes with the production of melanin (which causes sun and age spots) and is thought to stimulate the production of collagen and elastin. Since it is not overly emollient, it is beneficial for oily and blemish-prone skin. Aloe vera gel is a great alternative to a carrier oil for essential oil application. You can also find *aloe vera oil* if you are looking for increased moisturizing capabilities.

Essential Oils

Essential oils have been used to improve our lifestyles and health for thousands of years. You have probably used products with essentials oils, or a derivative of an essential oil, without even knowing it. Think of a cleaner with lemon oil added, Vicks® VapoRub™ which contains eucalyptus essential oil, or peppermints with peppermint oil to soothe an upset stomach.

Recently, essential oils are having their fifteen minutes of fame in the skincare world, and rightly so. Specific essential oils have anti-inflammatory, antibacterial, and antioxidant properties and promote circulation, improve the signs of aging, and help to heal skin conditions and damaged skin. They are truly skincare-ingredient powerhouses. But what exactly *are* they?

Essential oils are the tiny droplets of oil present between a plant's cells. Within this oil lies a critical component necessary for the plant's existence, which maintains its survival by attracting or warding off insects and animals. This is why plant oils may have a bright color, a favorable or strong smell, a bad taste, or even be poisonous. Some essential oils function by healing and protecting the plant physically. Therefore, essential oils are "essential" to a plant's existence.

The basic philosophy of human essential oil use: if these oils are so valuable as to aid in plants' survival, they should also help with our ailments.

Ancient doctors and practitioners began their own experiments, which developed (anecdotally) over many years into our current knowledge and application of essential oils. Even thousands of years ago, their valuable properties were tapped for use as medicines and practical treatments, such as insect repellants, dental hygiene, and elixirs for headaches, colds, muscle aches, nausea—the list goes on and on.

In skincare, essential oils were initially used in salves or carrier oils to heal wounds, infections, inflammation, and skin conditions. Today, the number of benefits has increased to include addressing dry skin, sun-damaged skin, wrinkles, excess oil production, and blemishes.

To best use essential oils in facial skincare, mix them with a carrier oil before applying. A carrier oil is an oil that dilutes and "carries" the essential oil to the cells below the skin's surface. This oil can be any oil listed in the facial oil section, or others that you research. It is easier to mix essential oils with a liquid oil, but they can be added to butters, fragrance-free creams, and aloe vera gel. As a general rule, add 3 – 7 drops to 0.5 ounce (1 tablespoon or 15 milliliters) of oil. Butters or creams will support a bit more essential oil: 6 – 15 drops to 0.5 ounce.

To avoid any possibility of irritation, start with the lowest-ratio mixture and observe how your skin reacts. **Never apply essential oils directly on your skin, except using Tea Tree Essential Oil as a spot treatment for blemishes**—besides possible irritation, most will evaporate before they have a chance to absorb.

Store your own essential oil and facial oil mixtures in small, dark-colored glass jars with roller balls or dropper tops, which can be found online or in stores that carry essential oil products. Or simply apply a drop or two of essential oil to a small amount of facial oil poured into the palm of your hand.

It is most important to choose quality essential oils, as many brands add synthetic ingredients or may even sell a fake product. Three keys to finding effective and pure essential oil brands are:

1. Look for small batch size, sometimes described as "hand-harvested," "small-batch," or "wild- crafted."
2. Look for USDA Certified Organic (although small companies may not be able to afford this certification process), or essential oils that are free of pesticides, synthetics, additives, or any adulteration.
3. Check out the company website for information regarding its history, practices, and whether they have independent lab testing of all their oils for purity and authentication.

Unfortunately, oil "grades" are only marketing jargon created by individual companies. So, watch out for "therapeutic grade," "pure grade," or "grade A" designations because, so far as quality goes, they mean nothing.

Listed below are *individual* essential oils and their skincare properties, but keep in mind there are exceptional skincare essential oil blends available in skincare products and as stand-alone essential oil products which are not listed here. Read the label and choose essential oil blends based on the mix of individual essential oils and their specific properties listed below.

For example, for problem skin, look for a blend containing tea tree oil; for premature aging skin, frankincense essential oil should be included; and for general skin health, search out carrot seed essential oil on the ingredient list.

One final tip: essential oils may be listed as "extracts" on the labels of finished products, such as moisturizers and serums.

Carrot Seed (*Daucus carota sativa*) is one of the best essential oils for skincare, as it treats a wide variety of skin issues effectively. It is regenerating, firming, and healing. Use it for wrinkle-prone, dry, acne and blemish-prone, hyperpigmented, and dull skin. It also treats rashes, rosacea, and burns. Note that carrot seed essential oil has a strong natural scent. Do not use during pregnancy.

Geranium, also known as **Rose Geranium**, (*Pelargonium graveolens*) is a skincare multi-tasker. It tones, revitalizes, and balances oil production. It is good for oily, dry, combination, acne or blemish-prone, and wrinkle-prone skin. Avoid during pregnancy.

Frankincense (*Boswellia carterii*) essential oil has been valued for centuries as a precious commodity, because its extraction method severely damages the tree it comes from, the Boswellia tree. Therefore, if you use it, please use sparingly. Some holistic estheticians claim it is the best essential oil for improving the signs of premature aging, and it also addresses inflammation. Do not use during pregnancy.

Rose, also known as **Rose Otto**, (*Rosa damascene*) is another treasured (and expensive) essential oil because of the enormous number of rose petals required to extract a small amount of essential oil. It is important to ensure the oil you choose is steam-distilled rather than extracted by a chemical solvent. The latter costs a lot less, but it is not recommended for skincare. Rose essential oil regenerates, firms, and heals the skin, making it ideal for wrinkle-prone, dry, sensitive, irritated, and inflamed skin.

German Chamomile, sometimes listed as **Blue Chamomile** or **Azulene** in products, (*Chamomilla recutita* or *Matricaria recutita*) is one of the best essential oils for inflammation. Its calming, soothing properties make it perfect for acne, rosacea, sensitive skin, inflammation, irritations, rashes, and sunburn.

Note: this oil is different than *Roman Chamomile* essential oil. Roman Chamomile is also good for the skin but does not have the same amazing anti-inflammatory properties.

Tea Tree (*Melaleuca alternifolia*) is probably the most well-known essential oil for skincare. It is fantastic to treat acne and blemishes as a drying spot treatment—this is the only essential oil I recommend applying directly onto the skin and *only for healing blemishes*. It can also be mixed with a carrier oil and used all over the face or affected areas. I use it in place of benzoyl peroxide, as it keeps the acid mantle in balance whilst achieving the same results, albeit over a slightly longer period of time. Tea Tree is also amazing for fighting infection without disrupting skin flora. These properties make it excellent for use on oily and/or acne and blemish-prone skin. Note that it has a strong, though not unpleasant, aroma.

Lavender (*Lavandula angustifolia*) is probably the most recognized, versatile, and popular essential oil for general use—and it is another skincare powerhouse. For oily and blemish-prone skin it is antibacterial, anti-inflammatory, and helps to balance oil production. It also treats dermatitis, eczema, and is great for sunburn because of its calming nature.

Sandalwood (*Santalum album*) is another popular skincare essential oil. It is significant because, along with its other properties (regenerating, revitalizing, antibacterial, anti-inflammatory, and healing), it is hydrating, making it great for dry and wrinkle-prone skin. It also works well on sensitive, oily, and blemish-prone skin.

Note: this essential oil is close to extinction (it is also used to treat wood furniture). Therefore, look for sandalwood grown in New Caledonia (in the South Pacific) where it is ethically harvested—for every tree that is cut, three are planted in its place.

Palmarosa (*Cymbopogon martini*) is a hydrating essential oil beneficial for all skin types, especially dry and wrinkle-prone skin. For acne-prone and oily skin, it is excellent at fighting infection, healing, and controlling the production of sebum. It also treats dermatitis and eczema.

Helichrysum (*Helichrysum italicum*) essential oil is expensive and rare, but one of my favorites. It is highly regenerating, healing, and is one of the best essential oils for sensitive skin—especially skin with rosacea, or skin that is susceptible to blood vessel dilation (also known as couperosis, where the skin remains red like a never-ending sunburn). It is also great for wrinkle and acne-prone skin. Mixed with an emollient carrier oil or appropriate cream, it helps fade circles under the eyes. And as a bonus, use Helichrysum to prevent or to heal stretch marks.

Essential Oil Hydrosols

Hydrosols may be the most versatile ingredient or stand-alone product in skincare and beyond.

Hydrosols are commonly made by collecting the steam byproduct produced when an essential oil is steam extracted. The steam turns to a liquid, and *voilá!*—an amazing tonic is created. Think of hydrosols as diluted, but still highly beneficial, forms of their corresponding essential oils. Therefore, for specific properties, see the essential oil list above.

In skincare, use a hydrosol in place of a toner, or mix it with a heavier cream or butter to make your own lotion (why buy a lotion that is filled with water when you can "make" one with a hydrosol?). To avoid the storage complications, just spray some hydrosol into your hand and mix in some cream at the time of use. You can also wipe off sweat after a workout with a saturated cotton round, or spray it on your face during an air flight to boost hydration. I also use my hydrosols as linen, pillow, and body sprays.

Because hydrosols contain water, they will "bloom"—meaning it will form solid substances that could be   mold or bacteria at the bottom of the container—when they are contaminated or get too old. Shelf life is between one to two years. It is best to keep larger bottles of hydrosol in your refrigerator and use a   smaller, dark glass container for daily use. Keep this smaller container in a dark, cool location.

Ingredients That Don't Fit in a Specific Category

Peptides are chains of amino acids that, when linked together, make up a protein. There are many   different types of peptides in skincare products, with two predominant categories.

The first are peptides purported to send messages to fibroblast cells to stimulate production of collagen—sometimes called "Regenerating Peptides." One specific peptide in this classification is rh- Oligopeptide, or EFG, and you will see it listed on labels as **Growth Factor**.

The second type of peptide claims to relax the muscles of the face to soften wrinkles—much like a   popular type of injection. These are sometimes named "Wrinkle Release Peptides."

Plant Stem Cells are the cells that keep the plant viable and protect it from harmful conditions— coincidentally sounding a lot like essential oils. Research shows these botanicals are super-powered antioxidants, believed to target the bottom layer of the epidermis where skin cells are created. They also   have the ability to protect these cells from UV ray damage, inhibit inflammation, neutralize free radicals,   and promote healthy cell production.[14] Other claims include improved skin cell longevity, increased skin   firmness, softened wrinkles, plumper skin, and increased hydration.

The most-studied plant stem cells are from grapeseed (*Vitis vinifera*), lemon verbena (*Verbascoside*),   apple (*Pyrus malus*), alpine rose (*Rhododendron ferrugineum*), and argan (*Argania spinosa*). These names should sound familiar: they are either oils, a fruit acid (AHA), or types of essential oils. Research has yet to show if we can reap the same benefits from these common forms of the botanical or whether it is best to reduce the ingredient down to a stem cell form. Time will tell.

Ceramides are lipids produced by our skin. They are natural moisturizers that form a protective barrier to prevent water loss. They also capture and bind water necessary for skin hydration. Topical ceramides are made from animals or plants and can serve the same purpose as our own naturally-occurring ceramides if we have dry, sensitive, rough, wrinkle-prone, and sun-damaged skin. Because our skin recognizes this substance, topical application is thought to work in coordination with our own skin ceramides— rendering it an effective skin barrier strengthener.

Collagen is a strong hydrator due to its ability to bind and retain many times its weight in water. It also acts as an emollient, forming a barrier on the skin to reduce moisture loss. **Collagen as a skincare ingredient does not penetrate and replenish the collagen we produce *in* our skin, but it is an effective ingredient for hydration, especially if you have dry skin.**

Elastin is similar to collagen but has a slightly different composition and is found in lower quantities in products. Though, like collagen, topical elastin cannot penetrate the skin and increase our own natural elastin volume, it can increase skin flexibility and tautness.

Ingredients to Avoid

Toxin-producers found in most commercially-made skincare products are of great concern to the public for three reasons:

1. There is an enormous amount of them in products with little regulation (the Food and Drug Administration typically pays little to no attention to skincare ingredients unless a huge safety issue becomes glaringly obvious over many years).
2. A large percentage of these toxin-producers penetrates all layers of the skin.
3. The toxins that penetrate go directly into your bloodstream without any organs, such as the liver, able to detoxify.

It is actually quite scary!

There are many books and internet articles naming and explaining the multitude of toxic ingredients in skincare. Since that is not the focus of this book, I won't elaborate beyond my top five(ish) list of what to absolutely avoid.

SD Alcohols including **Isopropyl Alcohol (Isopropanol), Methyl Alcohol (Methanol),** and **Ethyl Alcohol (Ethanol)** commonly referred to as **Rubbing Alcohol. Denatured Alcohol** is simply ethanol with additives to discourage consumption. Large corporate skincare products are *loaded* with alcohol (you can tell an ingredient is a type of alcohol because the word ends in "ol"), because it is cheap, and it can be used as a preservative. **Some alcohols are naturally-derived and are not considered harmful. A few of them are cetearyl alcohol, stearyl alcohol, cetyl alcohol, and benzyl alcohol, which may be present in some essential oils.**

The SD alcohols are very drying and strip the skin of its acid mantle. This action kills the skin flora we need for healthy skin. If your skin has acne, resist the urge to use products with SD alcohol even though it will temporarily dry out your blemishes. In the long run, you will disrupt your skin's own ability to fight off the bacteria that cause acne. It also causes dehydration because there is no longer a sebum barrier to hold in the moisture. If you like that tingly feeling you get after using a product that contains a SD alcohol, replace that product with one that includes AHAs or fruit enzymes.

Note: **Witch Hazel** found in drug stores is over 50 percent SD alcohols because, per government regulations, it must have a three-year shelf life; therefore, I consider it an alcohol. **Witch Hazel as an extract or hydrosol (*Hamamelis virginiana*) is a botanical**, wonderful for sunburns, skin irritations, and insect bites.

Benzoyl Peroxide will over-dry your skin and disrupt your skin flora balance leading to more problems. Tea tree oil mixed with aloe vera gel is a great substitute to help dry, oily skin. It may take more time to see results, but it will maintain the health of your skin long-term. Or try salicylic acid to reduce oiliness.

Mineral Oil, Petrolatum, and **Petroleum Jelly (Petrochemicals)** are derived from *petroleum*, the same substance that produces gasoline. It does start out as a natural product, but to make it palatable for skincare, it goes through a chemical process that changes its molecular structure (similar to how real food changes when it is processed). Petrochemicals can cause irritation, redness, clogged pores, and hives. You will find them in moisturizers and lip balm. It is also common to find them in topical medications prescribed by dermatologists.

Fragrances and **Perfumes** (sometimes listed as **parfum**) are snuck into every commercial skincare product, unless it is listed as "fragrance-free." Even "unscented" products have fragrances in them. And don't be fooled by the term "natural fragrances," because only 30 percent of that substance need be natural to bear that label. Over the years, I have seen many clients react with redness, rashes, and sensitivity from using products with fragrances or perfumes. Based on the sheer number of cases I've observed, I believe fragrances are one big cause of our sensitive skin epidemic. Fragrances and perfumes can also trigger nausea, headaches, dizziness, and coughing.[15] I only recommend products scented with pure essential oils, botanicals, herbs, or those listed as "fragrance-free," especially if you have sensitive skin.

Topical Steroids (a common one is **Hydrocortisone**) are found in many anti-itch products used to calm bug bites and allergic reactions. It is also found in many topical prescriptions used for skin conditions, such as dermatitis and eczema, as well as over-the-counter post-care treatments for use after a skin peel. **The problem lies in the fact that if you use a product containing a topical steroid for longer than a few days, it will make your condition worse.** It also causes a negative feedback loop where the more you use it, the more you need to use it, making it difficult to stop application. Then, once you stop using it, you will go through a withdrawal that can be very painful and itchy.

A few years ago, I developed dermatitis around my mouth and was prescribed a medication containing a topical steroid. I used it as directed (and made subsequent visits back to the dermatologist), but it just kept getting worse. It even traveled up around my nose and eventually went in my eyes. I was miserable, and my face was a red, itchy mess. **After a year of battling my dermatitis, I went "cold turkey" off the medication, used only aloe vera gel on my face after washing with a mild cleanser, and my face cleared up in just over two weeks.**

Now you can see why I get on my pedestal and preach against these medications. It is safe to use for a very short period of days (two to three), but there are other options that are healthier and have less risk of dependency and further irritation. If you suffer from a severe skin condition, you may want to see a traditional Chinese medicine doctor for a preparation that includes healing herbs.

And as far as treatment after a peel, any peel you receive should not be so harsh as to warrant use of a steroid to calm your skin. Trust your common sense and find a new esthetician if this is happening. If you receive a deeper peel from a dermatologist, however, it is more than likely he or she will prescribe an after-care medication containing a topical steroid. So, buyer beware!

To learn more about how to avoid toxic ingredients in skincare, I highly recommend The Environmental Working Group's Skin Deep database at: www.ewg.org/skindeep.

Now that you're up to speed on the most important and effective ingredients to look for in skincare, as well as a few to stay away from, let's learn how to best use them based on your skin type or condition.

Chapter Three: Skin Types and Conditions, and the Skincare Ingredients Best for Each

Dark spots, blemishes, and wrinkles, oh my! The truth is we all have skin issues we want to address (and if you don't, count yourself lucky!). The information in this chapter will empower you to address those issues based on your condition or skin type.

Note, it is not my intention to list every ingredient for two big reasons:

1. New ingredients are being tested and moved to market all the time, making it impossible to provide an up-to-date list.
2. There are many inactive ingredients mixed in a product to keep the ingredients from separating and to give it a nice consistency.

This abbreviated list will give you a good foundation for evaluating the active ingredients in your current and future products. These ingredients are also listed on the back of the skincare routine tear-out sheets found in the last chapter of this book.

Skin Types

Dry Skin

Dry skin does not produce enough sebum to create a barrier to effectively lessen moisture evaporation. Therefore, we need to add an outside hydrator and top it off with a moisturizer or oil to seal in the hydrator (moisture). Unfortunately, with dry skin, both the hydrator and moisturizer will absorb quickly into the skin making it necessary to reapply throughout the day—a tall task if you wear makeup.

One solution is to use a more emollient moisturizer or oil, which means you will need to try different ones so that you don't end up with a greasy look. If your skin looks dry (and possibly flaky), but does not respond well to a moisturizer (suddenly causing you to break out or experience clogged pores), you may have dehydrated skin. This means your skin is producing enough sebum, but there is a lack of underlying moisture. For this condition, try using a hydrating serum that contains a small amount of oil, drinking more water, and making sure your skin is protected from pollution and harsh weather—including windy days. Check out "An Amazing Hydration Trick" listed in *Chapter Four: Skincare Products,* as well. Also, keep in mind the biggest skin dehydrator of all is *smoking.*

Ingredients best for dry skin:

- **Avocado Oil**
- **Olive Oil**
- **Argan Oil** (a lighter oil, good for daytime application)
- **Coconut Oil**
- **Borage Seed Oil**
- **Squalane** (a lighter oil, good for daytime application)
- **Shea Butter**
- **All hydrators, but especially Hyaluronic Acid**
- **Collagen**
- **Elastin**
- **Ceramides**
- **Lactic Acid**
- **Malic Acid**

- **Vitamin E**
- **Rose Essential Oil and Hydrosol**
- **Sandalwood Essential Oil and Hydrosol**

Case Study: Linae

Linae came to me with rough, dry skin. So dry, in fact, that her face became flaky everyday even after using a moisturizer. She wanted to soothe her skin, but also wanted to her keep products down to a minimum. Because of the extreme nature of her skin, yet her desire to forgo a greasy look during the day, we needed to create a separate morning and night routine. A once a week exfoliating mask is also important for dry skin, because it helps with cell turnover and removes any dead skin flakes.

Morning:

1. Cleanse by wiping face with rose hydrosol and a cotton round.
2. Spray face with rose hydrosol. Do not wipe off.
3. Pat on a hydrating serum that contains hyaluronic acid. Do not skimp on the amount of serum. Try to "push" serum into skin.
4. Apply an emollient sunscreen.
5. Pat on eye cream.

Nighttime:

1. Cleanse and remove makeup with a gentle surfactant.
2. Spray face with rose hydrosol. Do not wipe off.
3. Apply hydrating serum as in the morning.
4. Apply vitamin E oil all over face.
5. Liberally apply a moisturizer that contains argan oil, avocado oil, honey, and ceramides.

6. Pat on eye cream.

Once a week:

Apply a homemade mask for 10 minutes that contains mashed pineapple, local honey, and lactic acid.

Nutritional Guidelines:

1. Drink 10 ounces of warm water first thing in the morning (a squeeze of lemon can be added). Wait 30 minutes before eating breakfast.
2. Increase water and herbal tea intake to half of body weight (measured in pounds) in ounces.
3. Increase omega-3 fatty acid intake via supplements (fish or krill oil) or food choices.

Oily Skin

I can relate to the trials of having very oily skin, having dealt with it for most of my life. Managing the almost constant sheen on my face has been a battle, to say the least. Also, with oily skin, you are more likely to have breakouts (especially after sweating) and larger pores. The good news is that your skin will look younger than your years as you age.

To address oiliness, make sure you exfoliate regularly and wash your face at least two times a day. Contrary to popular belief, you should not use products that overly dry your face, such as SD alcohol or hydrogen peroxide, as your skin will only produce more oil to counter the dryness. You do not want your oil ducts to go into overdrive.

The best ingredients for oily skin are slightly astringent, but do not contain alcohol. *Astringent* in this case means *constricting*—as in closing those pores a bit. Keep in mind, beneficial products and astringents should not sting or burn, with the exception of spa treatments in which an acid may be applied that creates a controlled stinging sensation. **Unfortunately, the astringent effect is only temporary, and pores cannot be permanently made smaller**–no matter what skincare companies claim. (See *Chapter Four: Skincare Products* for "The Best Treatment for Blackheads and Large Pores".) To prevent them from turning darker when the oil oxidizes in the pore (myth buster: that is not dirt clogging the pores), keep your face as clean as possible and use an astringent toner, hydrosol, and/or oil. Also, oil-blotting papers will become your best friend. I keep them everywhere so that I can use them throughout the day.

Ingredients best for oily skin:

- **All AHAs except Lactic Acid**
- **All Enzymes**
- **Salicylic Acid**
- **Retinol**
- **Charcoal**
- **Clays**
- **Moor Mud**
- **Squalane**
- **Hazelnut Oil**
- **Grapeseed Oil**
- **Calendula Oil**
- **Jojoba Oil**
- **Geranium Essential Oil and Hydrosol**
- **Tea Tree Essential Oil and Hydrosol**
- **Lavender Essential Oil and Hydrosol**

Case Study: Matt

Matt was concerned that his face looked like an "oil slick" (his words) half way into his day. He wanted his skin to look healthy but did not want to spend a lot of time tending to it.

Morning:

1. Cleanse with a mild gel facial cleanser.
2. Mix 2 to 3 drops of tea tree essential oil with a light liquid sunscreen and apply to face.

Mid-day:

Wipe face with tea tree hydrosol and a cotton round.

Nighttime:

1. Cleanse with a mild gel facial cleanser.
2. Mix 2 to 3 drops of tea tree essential oil with jojoba oil and apply to face.

Once a month:

Spa facial with an enzyme and AHA treatment and clay mask. (He said he would try his best to keep these appointments.)

Nutritional Guidelines:

1. Follow a high alkalinity diet.
2. Increase water and herbal tea intake to half of body weight (measured in pounds) in ounces.

Normal Skin

I don't think I've ever met a person who believes they have "normal" skin. But there is a range that falls under the umbrella of "normal." The best way to describe normal skin is: if at the end of the day, your skin is neither shiny with oil nor dry to the touch, and if most of the skin on your face is soft, moist, and has a healthy glow and color, then your skin is normal. It may lean oily (called "normal to oily") with larger pores and some shine in the T-zone, or lean dry (called "normal to dry") with dryer cheeks than the rest of your face.

The challenge for people with normal skin is to keep it that way. Weather, different seasons, age, toxins such as air pollution, sun exposure, a poor diet, and use of incorrect products can alter your skin and even cause a skin condition. It is important to reflect on these, especially if your skin has recently made a change for the worse. Also, preventative measures are always a good idea to ward off the effects of skin stressors—or at least delay inevitable changes, such as aging. A good start is to use sunscreen regularly, eat a healthy diet (more on this to come), and follow a consistent skincare practice.

If you have normal skin, there is more flexibility in choosing products. Any of the ingredients listed in this book, except those that are extremely emollient or drying, are appropriate. Just take into consideration an inclination towards oily or dry. Also, check out the ingredients listed below for combination skin.

Combination Oily and Dry Skin

Combination skin is a more intense version of "normal to oily" and "normal to dry," and can be tricky to treat. Should you apply products that focus on the dry areas or the oily areas? Do you need to buy two different products for the two different conditions of your skin? These questions can be answered based on the kind of combination skin you have.

The first type is normal skin that leans on the side of oily. If you take a quiz to determine your skin type, the result is only a generalization unless you neatly fit into a category. Normal skin can be a little bit dry, but not dry enough to be considered a dry skin type. And if the reverse is true, if skin is a bit oily, it will typically show up in the T-zone—oily forehead and nose (sometimes also on the chin and/or the   cheek area very close to the nose). This is probably a set state and your skin will continue to be this way   until you get older.

The key to this skin type is to use products for normal skin, with one or two as needed for the oily   areas. For example, you may choose to use a gentle oil or cream cleanser, with a more astringent oil or a   serum that doesn't contain oil. You can also add a product to address just the oily areas, such as an   astringent toner or tea tree hydrosol, especially if you tend to breakout or get blackheads in those areas.

Or the reverse may be the ticket—using a more aggressive cleanser, possibly containing salicylic acid or   AHAs, followed with a serum that contains oil. You may need to play around with what works best for   you. It is easy to get excessively concerned over the oily areas and use both very drying and exfoliating   products, but this is a mistake. It will lead to red, irritated, dehydrated skin that will now be classified as   "sensitive skin" in addition to being dry and oily (no fun). Instead, use appropriate products, and if you   are bothered by a shiny nose and forehead, use oil-blotting papers throughout the day.

The second kind of combination skin is one that is out of balance. This condition presents itself in   extremes—very oily forehead and nose with possible breakouts, and/or flaky, acutely dry cheeks. These opposite-ends-of-the-spectrum issues can result from using the wrong products for your skin over a long   period of time, over-exfoliating, neglecting your skin, or from a diet causing hormonal changes that affect   your skin. Then the stress of trying to deal with your skin problems causes more of the same.

The first thing to do is consider your diet. Have you been traveling a lot and eating more fast food than   usual? Have you been under a great deal of stress and unconsciously eating more processed snacks? See *Chapter Six: Skin Nutrition*, for simple ways to eat a more hormone-friendly diet with nutritious, skin- loving foods.

Second, consider if you are over-exfoliating. If the dry areas of your skin are red and sensitive, you may be overusing exfoliants—especially acids and retinol. Or, it may not be the frequency, but the percentage of acid or retinol is too high. If you have ruled out over-exfoliation, then you probably need to exfoliate more. Provided your skin is not sensitive, this is usually the best topical treatment you can do to balance out your skin. A facial or mild peel from a spa or esthetician school can jump-start this process, followed with a weekly mask or nightly acid or retinol serum. Or you can simply start out with the mask and/or the serum.

It is also a good idea to apply "middle-of-the-road" products which are not *too emollient* or *too drying* (think balance), until your skin evens out. Then you can see if you need to address the dryness or oiliness more.

Both kinds of combination skin types can benefit from using a hydrator along with a light moisturizer or oil. While it is apparent that the dry areas need moisture, remember that oily skin can also be dehydrated.

Specific ingredients that will help combination skin:

- If not sensitive, **Glycolic Acid, Retinol,** and **Lactic Acid** work best as exfoliators
- **Enzymes**
- **All Hydrators**
- **Squalane**
- **Hazelnut Oil**
- **Rice Bran Oil**
- **Marula Oil**
- **Cranberry Seed Oil**

- **Emu Oil**
- **Jojoba Oil**
- An appropriate **Essential Oil Skincare Blend** is especially beneficial, as it works to balance the skin
- **Carrot Seed Essential Oil and Hydrosol**
- **Geranium Essential Oil and Hydrosol**
- **Sandalwood Essential Oil and Hydrosol**
- **Palmarosa Essential Oil and Hydrosol**
- **Tea Tree Hydrosol** for oily areas

Case Study: Sarah

Sarah is a product junkie like me; but, unfortunately, her trying numerous different products to address her breakouts and fine lines around her eyes and lips led to her skin to become unbalanced. Her forehead was oilier than in the past, and the skin on her cheeks and chin was irritated and flaky. She applied an AHA and BHA serum every day as well as an acid-based mask once a week. This led to over-exfoliation and the dry, red skin combined with the skin on her forehead trying to overcompensate for the stripping of her sebum. We first worked on balancing her skin, and then addressed any concerns remaining after her skin normalized.

Morning:

1. Cleanse with a gentle gel cleanser.
2. Antioxidant serum containing magnesium ascorbyl phosphate (MAP), white tea, and jojoba oil.
3. Light, liquid sunscreen containing zinc oxide.
4. Until skin is balanced: apply hazelnut oil on cheeks and chin. Let absorb before applying makeup.

Nighttime:

1. Cleanse with a gentle gel cleanser.
2. Area treat breakouts with a BHA treatment when needed.
3. Once skin is balanced: retinol treatment. Let absorb before next step.
4. Hydrating serum containing hyaluronic acid and helichrysum hydrosol.
5. Hazelnut oil facial oil.

Once a month:

Home facial with a mask containing AHA and BHA followed by a soothing mask containing cucumber and aloe vera extract.

Nutritional Guidelines:

1. Follow a high alkalinity diet. Reduce processed food and sugar intake. Drink a *Simply Beautiful Skin* smoothie, containing fish collagen and hyaluronic acid, 5 mornings a week for breakfast.
2. Drink 10 ounces of warm water in the morning (a squeeze of lemon can be added). Wait 30 minutes before eating breakfast.
3. Increase water and herbal tea intake to half of body weight (measured in pounds) in ounces.
4. Take a probiotic supplement before bedtime and/or increase probiotic food choices.
5. Increase omega-3 fatty acid intake via supplements (fish or krill oil) or food choice.

Skin Conditions

Before we dive into the particular ingredients shown to improve skin conditions, I want to emphasize how important it is to first try to discover the root cause of your condition. This is best determined by looking at your diet, lifestyle, and stress level.

The foods we eat have an enormous effect on our skin, and I will talk about that in more detail in *Chapter Six: Skin Nutrition*. If you have a serious skin problem, I suggest you make an appointment with a nutritional esthetician, a dietician, or a nutritionist to create a healthy skin food plan.

Key to addressing any skin condition, and even specific types such as sensitive skin and skin that is aging prematurely, is to support our body's natural ability to heal and rejuvenate itself. Notice that I didn't mention seeing a dermatologist first. Dermatologists are great at what they do, but their standard philosophy is not to find the root cause of a condition. Instead, they usually focus on controlling the physical presentation—sometimes with aggressive measures.

I am not against doctor intervention—as I said before, I believe holistic care should include consideration of *all* treatments available. Sometimes no matter how much you clean up your diet, add lifestyle interventions, and use natural or over-the-counter treatments, your condition will stubbornly persist without an identifiable reason. In these cases, if your symptoms aggravate you enough to cause stress or interfere with your life, definitely see a medical professional. I simply want to emphasize the benefits of considering the least invasive, least toxic interventions first. And if you feel that a dermatologist visit is in your future, stress the importance to him or her of starting with the least aggressive treatment.

Hyperpigmented Skin

Pigmentation is the coloration of the skin by a substance called melanin. This pigment determines skin, eye, and hair color. It is also responsible for tans, which is a temporary discoloration. Sun spots, age spots, melasma (dark areas on the skin than can appear during pregnancy or other times of hormonal shifts), and dark spots left after pimples heal are considered hyperpigmentation. I consider them semi- permanent because, in most cases, you need to actively treat them with skin treatments, medication, or laser treatments to see the dark area fade or vanish.

Before we look at ingredients that help hyperpigmentation, let's explore the causes. Hyperpigmentation is triggered by five things:

1. Trauma–such as a blemish, causes irritation which leads to inflammation, initiating the skin's production of melanin to defend and protect the skin.
2. Inflammation—from an *external* cause, such as heavy pollution, excessive and repetitive heat, or wind burn; or an *internal* cause, such as a health condition, smoking, or eating a diet high in processed foods.
3. Hormones—when there is an imbalance of progesterone and estrogen in the body, melanocytes (the cells that produce melanin) are stimulated, causing more melanin to rise to the surface of the skin in an uneven distribution. Note that an unhealthy diet can cause hormone imbalances.
4. Sun exposure—stimulates melanin activity to protect the skin, resulting in a tan. This coloration protects you from more damage by the sun. However, this protection can go overboard and cause sun spots.
5. Free radical activity—causes melanin to be created to defend the damaging effects.

There are three ways to address hyperpigmented skin, and I bet you can guess the first one:

1. Prevent as much trauma, inflammation, sun exposure, and free radical damage as you can. Considering skincare specifically, this means applying sunscreen and antioxidant-rich products regularly. For best results from using products with any of the ingredients listed below, you must be almost obsessive with your use of sunscreen, including on cloudy days and in reapplying throughout the day.
2. Use products that contain ingredients that inhibit the melanin production or distribution process.
3. Use products that contain ingredients that treat the dark spots (and some ingredients do both).

Note: some people find laser treatments are the most effective and quickest way to remove dark spots. But keep in mind that laser treatments are costly and can cause hypopigmentation (all melanin is removed from the area leading to white spots). Hypopigmentation cannot be treated; you just have to hope that over time the white spots, with exposure to the sun, will blend in with the color of the rest of your skin.

Preventative ingredients:

All Antioxidant and Sunscreen Ingredients (see *Chapter Four: Skincare Products* for sunscreen information).

Hydroquinone is probably the most controversial ingredient we will cover. The controversy stems from hydroquinone being banned in South Africa many years ago; but it was found that the banned product was adulterated with mercury and other dangerous contaminants, which was likely the reason for the harmful side effects.[16] Another source of concern is that with extended continuous use, it has been shown to cause ochronosis, a darkening of the skin, in darker skin tones—the exact opposite of the desired effect.

However, it is the best preventative and treatment available for uneven skin tone due to hyperpigmentation, because it is the most effective ingredient to inhibit melanin production. It also acts as a skin brightener and lightener. For the best and safest results, use every night, stop using after four months, and cycle its use with other ingredients listed below (note: it may take two to three months to see any improvement). Retail products go up to 2 percent concentration, but using a medically prescribed 4 percent solution, along with a retinol product, will be most effective. If you are concerned about the safety of hydroquinone, keep in mind that the natural ingredients **Bearberry Extract, Mulberry, White Mulberry,** and **Arbutin** will break down into hydroquinone when they are absorbed into the skin.

Kojic Acid is derived from mushrooms and other fungi and is used to naturally prevent fruits from turning brown. It has a similar effect as hydroquinone, although not as potent and quick-acting. It is an effective lightening agent.

Licorice Extract is another natural melanin inhibitor. It may also even out your skin tone by lightening dark spots.

Gigawhite is a compound of seven different extracts from Swiss alpine plants. This combination has been found exceptional in preventing melanin production. Also, it may lighten dark areas.

Treatments—these ingredients either encourage sloughing off of the top layer of darkened skin cells or have been found to lighten dark spots, or both:

- **Glycolic Acid**
- **Mandelic Acid**
- **Azelaic Acid (or Azeloyl Glycine)**

- **Retinol**
- **Avocado Oil**
- **Carrot Seed Essential Oil**

Case Study: Remy

Remy was concerned with dark spots on her face and décolleté caused by sun damage and age. She chose not to go the route of seeking out medical or laser treatment. We developed a regime to lighter and brighten her skin naturally. Her skin also leaned on the dry side. Products, with the exception of cleanser and eye gel, were applied on her face, neck and upper chest area.

Morning:

1. Cleanse with a creamy cleanser.
2. Geranium hydrosol as a toner.
3. Antioxidant and brightening serum containing vitamins green tea extract and licorice extract.
4. Sunscreen.
5. Eye gel.

Nighttime:

1. Makeup remover.
2. Creamy cleanser.
3. Geranium hydrosol.
4. Retinol treatment. Let absorb before next step.
5. Brightening and hydrating serum containing arbutin, kojic acid, and hyaluronic acid.
6. A fragrance-free avocado oil moisturizer mixed with 2 – 3 drops of carrot seed oil.

7. Eye gel.

Once a week:

Apply a mask containing AHAs, lactic acid, and glycolic acid.

Nutritional Guidelines:

1. Follow a high alkalinity diet. Reduce sugar intake and increase food choices high in antioxidants.
2. Drink 10 ounces of warm water in the morning (a squeeze of lemon can be added). Wait 30 minutes before eating breakfast.
3. Increase water and herbal tea intake to half of body weight (measured in pounds) in ounces

Sensitive Skin

The amount of people reporting sensitive skin has been on the rise for several years. This may be due to exposure to harsh elements or products rather than an innate skin type. Sun exposure, pollution, a harsh climate, as well as overuse of exfoliators and products with added fragrances and colors can lead to sensitivity and even to skin conditions, such as rosacea.

The best rule of thumb for sensitive skin is "less is more"—perfect for a simplified skincare routine! This advice is ironic, since there are many helpful ingredients for sensitive skin. Keep in mind that any of them would work depending on what purpose you want them to serve—you should not try to use them all.

This is another skin condition that benefits from sunscreen use; just make sure you use a physical sunscreen rather than a chemical, because they are gentler on the skin. Zinc oxide is the best physical sunscreen for sensitive skin. Also, do not apply retinol, enzymes, or acids (except those noted below) as they could exacerbate the situation. It is very important not to use products with any fragrances, perfumes, detergents, or harsh preservatives, because they are known skin irritants. **Look for products listed as "fragrance-free." In addition, choose pure products with the least amount of ingredients.**

If your skin has become extremely sensitized to any product you apply, limit what you use to only water, helichrysum hydrosol (*pat* on with a cotton round), and a pure oil. (I recommend either sea buckthorn oil, evening primrose oil, or avocado oil in this case.) Use a physical sun protectant, such as a hat, every time you go outdoors. Stay with this regime for approximately two weeks to, hopefully, calm your skin. After this period, add one product at a time, and see if your skin reacts. When you add a product, make sure it is a product with very few ingredients (especially preservatives), and that it doesn't contain any added fragrances, perfumes, or colors. Consider trying a sunscreen with zinc oxide and aloe vera gel early in your product trials.

<u>Ingredients best for sensitive skin:</u>

- **Seaweed Extract** comes in many different types and colors including coral, blue, and brown. In a product, such as a serum, you will usually find a combination. This marine extract is very soothing and hydrating. It moisturizes and protects the skin by forming a gentle protective gel on the surface of the skin and is packed with vitamins and minerals. It may also be listed as **"Aldavine."**
- **Sea Whip** is another marine-derived ingredient extracted from a creature that lives in coral reefs. It has been found to have superior anti-inflammatory and healing properties due to its ability to neutralize an enzyme responsible for skin irritation. It is very soothing and calming.
- **Allantoin** is a botanical extract from the comfrey plant that is healing, calming, and soothing. It is believed to stimulate new tissue growth and help heal damaged skin.
- **Chamomile** and **Yarrow** (sometimes listed as **Bisabolol**) are both botanicals known for their anti- inflammatory and soothing properties.
- **Aloe Vera Extract or Gel**
- **Green Tea Extract**
- **All Hydrators**
- **Vitamin C, only in the form of Magnesium Ascorbyl Phosphate**
- **Papaya (Papain) Enzyme**
- **Azelaic Acid (Azeloyl Glycine)**
- **Mandelic Acid**
- **Malic Acid**
- **Borage Seed Oil** (especially if dry and sensitive)
- **Chamomile**
- **Sea Buckthorn Oil**
- **Rice Bran Oil**
- **Evening Primrose Oil**

- **Hemp Seed Oil**
- **Jojoba Oil**
- **Shea Butter**
- **Zinc Oxide**
- **Ceramides**
- **Helichrysum Essential Oil and Hydrosol**
- **German Chamomile Essential Oil**
- **Chamomile Hydrosol**
- **Carrot Seed Essential Oil and Hydrosol**

Case Study: Jasmine

Jasmine has reactive skin (skin that turns bright red like a blush when new or strong products are applied, when she is in cold or windy weather, or when she gets overheated). Reactive skin cannot be changed. She also has fair skin which is susceptible to both sensitive skin and rosacea. Her skin had become red and irritated, especially on her cheeks. She wanted to reduce these symptoms before she potentially develops rosacea.

Morning:

1. Very gentle gel cleanser.
2. Spray face with a combination solution of helichrysum and chamomile hydrosol. Do not wipe off.
3. Pat on antioxidant serum containing magnesium ascorbyl phosphate (MAP).
4. Sunscreen containing zinc oxide.

Nighttime:

1. Very gentle gel cleanser.
2. Spray face with a combination solution of helichrysum and chamomile hydrosol. Do not wipe off.

3. Pat on serum containing seaweed extract, aloe vera gel, bisabolol, glycerin, green tea extract, allantoin, and German chamomile essential oil.
4. Pat on hemp seed oil.

After a workout:

Hold a face wipe made for sensitive skin on face for a moment. (Homemade wipe: cotton rounds soaked in aloe vera juice and appropriate hydrosol such as chamomile.) Pat sweat off, if present.

Monthly:

Soothing spa facial with papaya enzyme and azelaic acid treatments.

Nutritional Guidelines:

1. Follow an elimination diet to determine any food sensitivities.
2. Drink 10 ounces of warm water in the morning (a squeeze of lemon can be added). Wait 30 minutes before eating breakfast.
3. Increase water and herbal tea intake to half of body weight (measured in pounds) in ounces.
4. Take a probiotic supplement before bedtime and/or increase probiotic food choice.
5. Drink 1 ounce of aloe vera gel before bedtime.

Acne/Blemish-Prone Skin

Acne seems to be a cruel trick the universe plays on many of us, striking mainly where people look at us   most—our face. It is worst during the teen years when we are trying to build our confidence and self- presence. And for some us, it continues through our 30's, 40's, and beyond (I have battled it for most of my life). Appropriate skincare will definitely help, but medical intervention may be necessary for some types of acne.

Acne can be caused by hormones; internal inflammation; overabundance of harmful bacteria in either or both the skin and intestinal microbiome; stress; sweat; and humidity; or any combination thereof.

There are three types of acne: Comedonal, Papular/Pustule, and Cystic.

Comedonal consists of blackheads and whiteheads without redness or irritation. This type is caused by excess oil pooling in pores and becoming oxygenated. When this oil is oxygenated it turns dark (blackheads are not caused by dirt). A whitehead is just a blackhead with skin that has grown over the clogged pore.

The second type, and the most common, is Papular/Pustule acne where the clogged pore has now been infected with the bacteria *P. acnes*. Pink or red inflamed bumps filled with puss are present.

The third type, Cystic, is a serious condition of hard, painful, and sometimes very large bumps under the skin.

Acne or blemish-prone skin type routines are the most difficult to keep simple. Because it is the most common skin issue, many helpful practices have been found to keep breakouts to a minimum.

Practices to consider for acne and blemishes:

- o Wash your face at least twice a day (some people may need a mid-day wash also) and after you work out or sweat.
- o Wash your hair often and, if you use conditioner, wash your face (or any part of your body affected by acne) after you rinse off the conditioner.

o   Do not use a mechanical scrub or brush. This may be too harsh on your face and cause the harmful *P.acnes* bacteria to spread.

o   Do not touch your face AT ALL (yes, in CAPS!), except during your skincare routine.

o   Change your pillowcases frequently.

o   Do not rub your face on pet hair.

o   As far as the facial oils listed below, use only a very small amount. Some serums have a very little bit of oil in them and that would be sufficient.

o   For essential oil application, try using aloe vera gel as a carrier instead of an oil.

o   For an exfoliator, stay away from lactic acid as it is too hydrating.

o   Maintain your skin flora by never using antibacterial soap or benzoyl peroxide and by applying the   "DIY Probiotic Skin Balancing Mask" (recipe found in *Chapter Four: Skincare Products*) or honey as a mask once a week. Do not purchase "probiotic lotions"—at this time, they don't work (the lotion needs to include a preservative, and preservatives kill the good bacteria).

o   As best you can, follow the dietary guidelines found in *Chapter Six: Skin Nutrition*, because food can make a huge difference in acneic skin. In a nutshell, increase probiotic food in your diet, drink lots of water, cut out dairy foods, decrease sugar intake as much as possible, and take in more good oils like coconut and olive.

o   Medical spa treatments include weekly acne facials, blue light treatments, and laser treatments   designed to kill *P. acnes* bacteria and lessen the appearance of acne scars. See a medical esthetician for a personalized treatment plan.

o   Do not feel like a failure if you try everything and you still have breakouts. Medical intervention may be necessary, at least in the short term. One of the most common treatments for acne is antibiotics. If you and your medical professional decide this is the best course of action, increasing your probiotic intake will help balance your intestinal flora (antibiotics kill all bacteria, including the beneficial bacteria). Once your course of antibiotics is complete, decrease your intake slowly and beware of a rebound effect. This means that your acne may get worse before it gets better. Give it at least a week off of the antibiotics to discern the true condition of your skin.

Before we get into the beneficial ingredients for acne, I want to talk about a popular acne ingredient you should definitely avoid: benzoyl peroxide.

Benzoyl peroxide works very well on comedonal and papular/pustule acne initially. However, it is so drying that it disrupts or destroys the natural flora (good bacteria) located on the skin. This is counterproductive as you need that flora to fight the harmful bacteria (*P. acnes*). So, over time you will actually be helping *P. acnes* proliferate, making it almost impossible to get under control. Also, using an ultra-drying product like this sends a signal to your pores to produce more oil. This starts a snowball effect, where the more you use benzoyl peroxide, the more you will need it.

Apply salicylic acid and tea tree extract or oil instead of benzoyl peroxide.

Ingredients best for acne and blemish-prone skin:

- **Salicylic Acid**, which also can be listed as **Willow Bark** or **BHA**, has been described in the exfoliation section of this chapter, but bears repeating: this is the best treatment ingredient for acne—hands down. It dissolves the impactions that can create up pimples and reduces the production of sebum. You can find it in cleansers, toners, and treatment serums. Monitor how your skin responds to one or two products containing salicylic acid. If all your products contain it, you may end up with flaky skin. Also, keep in mind that you may need to adjust the number of salicylic acid-containing products you use during different times of the month and stressful periods, and depending on the weather and how often you perspire.

- **Tea Tree Oil and Hydrosol** have also been previously described in the essential oil section of this chapter. Tea tree oil and hydrosol are the best substitutes for benzoyl peroxide. In studies, tea tree oil has been found to work as well as benzoyl peroxide (however, it does take longer to see results) without the negative side effects.[17]

- **Charcoal** (I like **Activated Coconut Charcoal**) is usually found in masks. There are also charcoal cleansing bars on the market, but I generally do not recommend them as they may be too drying, which in turn will knock your skin flora out of balance. Charcoal is super absorbent and draws out impurities and excess oil. It is also antibacterial, healing, anti-inflammatory, purifying, and helps prevent future breakouts.

- **Clays** are also mostly used in cleansing bars or masks and can be purchased as stand-alone products in powder form to make your own masks (mix with water or tea tree hydrosol). There are a multitude of different types of clays. The best for acne is **French Green Clay,** as it is excellent for drawing impurities and toxins out of the skin. It is very drying, so do not use on sensitive skin. For sensitive skin, choose **Kaolin Clay** (including yellow and red), also called **China Clay**, and **Rose Clay**. For a mineral boost, choose **Sea Clay** or **Dead Sea Clay**.

- **Moor Mud** is a relatively unknown ingredient that is highly beneficial to blemish-prone skin. It is healing, anti-inflammatory, detoxifying, and astringent (tightens pores). It is also great at   drawing out impurities. Like clay, you will find this ingredient in masks, or purchase separately and you can make your own mask.

- **Apple Cider Vinegar** (if you can stand the smell!) kills harmful bacteria while allowing your acid   mantle to remain in balance. You can use this as a toner to remove any excess dirt or makeup   post-cleansing and prepare the skin for treatment serums without over-drying the skin. **It is best to cut straight apple cider vinegar with water and/or hydrosols. Try one-part vinegar and four- parts water and/or hydrosol before applying.**

- **Retinol**
- **Azelaic Acid**
- **Neem Oil**
- **Jojoba Oil**
- **Hemp seed Oil**
- **Calendula Oil**
- **Aloe Vera Extract or Gel**
- **Zinc Oxide**
- **Carrot Seed Essential Oil and Hydrosol**
- **Sandalwood Essential Oil and Hydrosol**
- **Palmarosa Essential Oil and Hydrosol**
- **Lavender Essential Oil and Hydrosol**

Case Study: Michael

Michael has suffered from breakouts over his entire face for a few years. He tried a   nationally advertised, popular skincare program to treat acne, and it worked for a   short time. Then his acne became worse. This experience soured his desire to adhere to an overly involved program. He followed the following skincare regime and dietary advice, and his breakouts lessened a great deal. However, he was not satisfied   with these results and decided to seek out medical advice, rather than electing to receive a weekly acne facial or begin laser or light therapy.

Morning:

1. Cleanse with a cleanser that contains salicylic acid.
2. Apply light, liquid sunscreen that contains zinc oxide.

Mid-day and after a workout:

Pat face with a commercially-made apple cider vinegar and hydrosol wipe.

Nighttime:

1. Cleanse with a cleanser that contains salicylic acid.
2. Apply a salicylic acid and retinol treatment. Let absorb before next step.
3. Spray face with tea tree hydrosol. Do not wipe off.
4. Lightly apply neem oil.

Nutritional Guidelines:

1. Drink 10 ounces of warm water in the morning (a squeeze of lemon can be added). Wait 30 minutes before eating breakfast.
2. Increase water and spearmint tea intake to half of body weight (measured in pounds) in ounces.
3. Remove all dairy from diet, except very hard cheeses.
4. Limit fast food intake to once a week or less.
5. Increase omega-3 fatty acid intake in the form of supplements (fish or krill oil) or food choice.
6. Greatly reduce sugar intake. Try to limit to fruits with skin present.
7. Increase gamma linolenic acid (GLA) intake by adding borage seed oil and spirulina to daily smoothie.

8. Take a probiotic supplement before bedtime.
9. Take a probiotic supplement before bedtime and/or increase probiotic food   choice.

Possible Rosacea

Like sensitive skin, rosacea diagnoses are on the rise. In fact, you may have rosacea and not even know   it, because it appears as sensitive skin—often with what resemble acne blemishes—and gradually gets worse if not treated. One way to tell (note: contact a health professional for a diagnosis), is if your face   is flushing more and the blemishes you have are small and contain transparent liquid. However, you   don't need to have blemishes to have rosacea; many people experience dry, flaky, red skin.

There are three types of rosacea for purposes of medical diagnosis, but I am going to separate   beneficial ingredients by these two varieties: oily, pustule-prone; and dry, sensitive.

Like acne-prone skin, there are several lifestyle practices that will help your condition. However, just like   with acne, you may need to seek medical advice depending on the severity of your condition.

Helpful practices for possible rosacea:

o *Be gentle on your skin! "More is not better" with this condition. Choose products with the   least amount of ingredients; or choose to use pure oils, essential oils, or hydrosols on their   own.*
o **Do not use products with fragrances, perfumes, detergents, or harsh preservatives. Look for   "fragrance-free" labeling.**
o Be wary of tretinoin prescriptions because they may be too harsh and make the situation worse.
o Salicylic acid and essential oils can be very helpful, but start with a very low percentage.
o Do not use mechanical exfoliation, such as scrubs or brushes.

o   Stay away from glycolic and lactic acid.
o   Do not use any skin treatments with SD alcohol (or its derivatives), peppermint, menthol, or   benzoyl peroxide.
o   Eat probiotic foods and apply the "DIY Probiotic Skin Balancing Mask" (recipe found in *Chapter   Four: Skincare Products*) or a honey mask once a week. Probiotics will lessen redness and   increase skin barrier strength resulting in less stinging, burning, and dryness.
o   A change in your diet could make an enormous difference (see *Chapter Six: Skin Nutrition*).
o   Use sunscreen ALL THE TIME (you know I'm serious when I use CAPS), even in cloudy weather or   if you will be indoors all day. The only exception is when you're sleeping you may go without.

Reapply throughout the day.

o   Try removable car screens. These are a screen on one side with a plastic wrap-type covering on   the other and are great for the side windows of your car.
o   If needed, refrain from intense workouts for a while, especially if they are done in a heated   room.
o   When you finish a sweaty workout, make sure you pat your face (don't rub) with a face wipe or   cotton round that contains aloe or an appropriate essential oil hydrosol.
o   If you experience blemishes with your rosacea, look over the acne/blemish-prone skin section. Many of these tips will help; just be mindful of your sensitive skin and be gentle with it.
o   If you have deep flushing, laser treatment is very effective. The two laser therapies I have seen   best results with are IPL (Intense Pulse Light) and PDL (Pulsed Dye Laser). You will most likely   need a series of treatments, usually three to six, spaced about a month apart. Make sure you   seek out a medical esthetician who is experienced in working with

clients with rosacea. There is an art to these treatments and, unfortunately, a basic laser treatment may make your condition worse.

o   Like dealing with acne, if you try everything listed here and *still* have a problem, you may need to seek medical help. Some traditional medical interventions can be very harsh on skin with rosacea, such as tretinoin (Retin A®). I do not recommend this treatment. However, if you are experiencing breakouts, you and your medical professional may decide that a course of antibiotics is the next step. Increase your probiotic intake to help balance your intestinal flora (antibiotics kill all bacteria—including the beneficial bacteria). Also, once it is decided that you should discontinue antibiotics, decrease your intake slowly and beware of a rebound effect. This means your breakouts may get worse before they get better. Give it at least a week off of the antibiotics to discern the true condition of your skin.

If your skin has become extremely sensitized to any product you apply, limit what you use to only water, helichrysum hydrosol (*pat* on with a cotton round), and a pure oil. (I recommend either calendula, sea buckthorn oil, evening primrose oil, or avocado oil in this case.) Use a physical sun protectant, such as a hat, every time you go outdoors. Stay with this regime for approximately two weeks to, hopefully, calm your skin. After this period, add one product at a time, and see if your skin reacts. When you add a product, make sure it is a product with very few ingredients (especially preservatives), and that it doesn't contain any added fragrances, perfumes, or colors. Consider trying a sunscreen with zinc oxide and aloe vera gel early in your product trials.

Oily/Pustule-Prone Possible Rosacea Ingredients:

- **Vitamin C in the form of Magnesium Ascorbyl Phosphate (MAP)**
- **Salicylic Acid** (start with lower percentages)
- **Mandelic Acid**
- **Papaya (Papain) Enzyme**
- **Azelaic Acid (or Azeloyl Glycine)**
- **Green Tea Extract**
- **Allantoin**

- **Jojoba Oil**
- **Rice Bran Oil**
- **Calendula Oil**
- **Zinc Oxide**
- **Helichrysum Essential Oil and Hydrosol**
- **German Chamomile Essential Oil**
- **Tea Tree Essential Oil and Hydrosol**
- **Carrot Seed Essential Oil and Hydrosol**
- **Frankincense Essential Oil and Hydrosol**
- **Lavender Essential Oil and Hydrosol**
- **Aloe Vera Gel** (especially as a carrier for essential oil)

Dry/Flaky Possible Rosacea Ingredients:

- **All Hydrators**
- **Vitamin C in the form of Magnesium Ascorbyl Phosphate (MAP)**
- **Mandelic Acid**
- **Papaya (Papain) Enzyme**
- **Azelaic Acid**
- **Green Tea Extract**
- **Allantoin**
- **Shea Butter**
- **Sea Buckthorn Seed Oil**
- **Ceramides**
- **Zinc Oxide**
- **Helichrysum Essential Oil and Hydrosol**
- **Chamomile Hydrosol**
- **German (Blue) Essential Oil and Hydrosol**
- **Carrot Seed Essential Oil and Hydrosol**
- **Rose Essential Oil and Hydrosol**

- **Frankincense Essential Oil and Hydrosol**

Case Study: Me!

My latest, among many, skin problem is oily/pustule-prone rosacea. I now have it under control, but initially I was a red-faced, blemished mess. I have fair skin with an ethnic background (mostly northern European) predisposed to acquire rosacea. Also, I admit to formerly overusing exfoliating products (see my love for exfoliators in the second chapter). I learned my lesson, and along with other interventions, I only exfoliate with a low-percentage level retinol treatment (now that the rosacea is under control), a daily area-specific and appropriate AHA treatment, and a monthly facial for skin with rosacea.

Morning:

1. Cleanse with a gentle gel cleanser.
2. Pat skin with a mixture of helichrysum and chamomile hydrosol.
3. Antioxidant serum with magnesium ascorbyl phosphate (MAP).
4. Light, liquid sunscreen with zinc oxide.

After a yoga class:

Pat face with a cotton ball saturated with helichrysum and chamomile hydrosol. If it is hot weather, I let the air-conditioner in my car blow on my face briefly.

Nighttime:

1. Cleanse with a gentle gel cleanser.
2. Pat skin with hydrosol mixture.

3. Apply a serum on my forehead (where my pustules appear) containing azeloyl glycine (a form of azelaic acid) and mandelic acid.
4. Apply a low-percentage level retinol treatment (only after rosacea is under control). Let absorb before next step.
5. Pat on a mixture of argan, rosehip seed, and calendula oil.

Nutritional Guidelines:

1. Follow a high alkalinity diet. Reduce processed food and sugar intake. *Simply Beautiful Skin* smoothie, containing fish collagen and hyaluronic acid, 5 mornings a week.
2. Drink 10 ounces of warm water in the morning (a squeeze of lemon can be added). Wait 30 minutes before eating breakfast.
3. Increase water and herbal tea intake to half of body weight (measured in pounds) in ounces.
4. Avoid dairy, red wine, and spicy foods.
5. Take a probiotic supplement before bedtime.
6. Drink 1 ounce of aloe vera gel before bedtime, until rosacea is under control.

Premature Aging Skin

The term "anti-aging," used throughout the skincare industry, is a serious pet peeve of mine—and I'm not alone. *Allure* magazine has agreed to ban this term from their publication, per their September 2017 cover.

First of all, the term doesn't even make sense—we are all aging if we are living. Secondly, it is another unattainable term skincare companies have imposed on us. **Our skin will age, and nothing we put on it, no matter how expensive, exclusive, or of the latest technology, is going to change that.**

The reality is, as we age, our skin becomes thinner because cell turnover decreases; it becomes drier and less hydrated because we produce less sebum and hyaluronic acid in the skin; it takes longer to repair itself due to a decrease in our skin barrier integrity; and we produce less collagen and elastin, so our skin is less plump and springy.

Unfortunately, we cannot erase deep wrinkles and lift sagging skin with skincare products alone. But hope is not lost! There is plenty we can do to improve the health of our skin to stave off the signs of aging as long as possible. If you spent too much time in the sun when you were younger, as I did (even using tin foil to speed up my tan–yikes!), there are ingredients that will brighten and even out our skin tone, smooth out the texture, and soften wrinkles. **Retinol** (or if you go the prescription route: tretinoin) is the closest ingredient we have to a miracle worker, as it can address all of those goals effectively. See *Chapter Two: Skincare Ingredients* for more information. In addition, check out two more skincare ingredients described in Chapter Two–**peptides and plant stem cells.** Both have attributes advantageous for individuals interested in reducing the signs of aging in the skin, such as lessen wrinkling, plumping the skin, and increasing skin firmness and regeneration of skin cells. Also, I never miss an opportunity to tout a personal favorite of mine, **frankincense essential oil**–known to tighten the skin, boost rejuvenation, and protect it from free radicals, among many other attributes. And, as mentioned earlier, free radical activity is the number one cause of skin aging, so every day apply a product containing an **antioxidant,** and never forget the most important preventative measure: **sunscreen.**

Nutrition has a lot to do with how our skin ages. See *Chapter Six: Skin Nutrition* for details, but forewarning—sugar is not your friend. Also, maintaining your skin flora with probiotics in your diet, and applying a weekly probiotic mask, such as the "DIY Probiotic Skin Balancing Mask" (recipe found in *Chapter Four: Skincare Products*) or a plain yogurt mask that includes probiotic strains of bacteria, will help hydrate the skin and lessen sun damage. In addition, studies show a probiotic mask may increase collagen production.[18]

Since skin that is aging prematurely can have varying needs depending on the person, check out other sections in this chapter for additional tips and recommendations. For example, to focus on specific objectives such as evening out skin tone or helping dry skin, review the hyperpigmented or dry skin sections, respectively.

Ingredients that directly address wrinkle-prone, premature aging skin:

- **All Hydrators listed, but especially Hyaluronic Acid**
- **All Antioxidants listed, but especially Green Tea Extract, Resveratrol, and Vitamin E (best combined with Vitamin C)**
- **Retinol** (start with a low-percentage product, increase the percentage as your skin acclimates)
- **Glycolic Acid**
- **Lactic Acid**
- **Mandelic Acid**
- **Argan Oil**
- **Rosehip Seed Oil**
- **Cranberry Seed Oil**
- **Collagen**
- **Elastin**
- **Peptides (Growth Factor)**
- **Plant Stem Cells**
- **Geranium Essential Oil and Hydrosol**
- **Rose Essential Oil and Hydrosol**
- **Frankincense Essential Oil and Hydrosol**

Case Study: Kate

Kate is a woman in her late 50s who began taking care of her skin in earnest about 15 years ago. When she was younger, sunscreen not promoted, and tanning was popular. Fine lines and sagging along her chin line has begun to bother her.

Although she doesn't have much hyperpigmentation, she would like to even out her skin tone and help her skin to look healthier. She tried Retin-A® when her dermatologist prescribed it, but she found it too drying. Her skin leans on the dry side; however, it is not overly dry as can be common with prematurely aging skin. She is concerned with the signs of aging on her neck and décolleté; therefore, products are applied to these areas also.

Morning:

1. Cleanse with a gel cleanser.
2. Antioxidant serum with vitamins C and E.
3. Sunscreen.
4. Pat on eye cream.

Nighttime:

1. Cleanse with a gel cleanser.
2. Retinol treatment. Let absorb before next step.
3. "Anti-aging" serum containing peptides and plant stem cells.
4. DIY facial oil containing argan oil, cranberry oil, rosehip seed oil, and frankincense essential oil.
5. Pat on eye cream.

Once a week:

Apply an exfoliating mask for 20 minutes that contains glycolic and mandelic acid.

Nutritional Guidelines:

1. Follow a high alkalinity diet. Reduce processed food intake.
2. Drink a *Simply Beautiful Skin* smoothie, containing fish collagen and hyaluronic acid, at least 5 mornings a week.
3. Remove most refined sugar and simple carbohydrates from diet.
4. Drink 10 ounces of warm water in the morning (a squeeze of lemon can be added). Wait 30 minutes before eating breakfast.
5. Increase water and herbal tea intake to half of body weight (measured in pounds) in ounces.
6. Increase omega-3 fatty acid intake via supplements (fish or krill oil) or food choice.
7. Take a probiotic supplement before bedtime and/or increase probiotic food choice.

Dark Circles Under the Eyes

- **Vitamin K** is one of the best ingredients for under-eye circles because of its ability to reduce blood flow to the skin.
- **Retinol** (make sure it is a low percentage) increases collagen production and rebuilds thin skin.
- **Helichrysum Essential Oil** in a carrier oil.
- **Kojic Acid** and **Licorice Extract** are both lightening agents.

Eye Puffiness

- **Matrixyl 3000** is found in many eye products. It consists of peptides that stimulate the production of collagen and regulate cell activity, which leads to repairing and rejuvenating the skin.

- **Niacinamide** is soothing, healing, and helps to repair the skin barrier. It works fast to reduce   redness and inflammation.
- **Caffeine** stimulates the skin while also tightening and firming.
- **Cucumber Extract** is cooling and soothing. It is also rich in vitamin C.
- **Chilled Aloe Gel** is my favorite to reduce puffiness from my eyes. Pat this on to soothe and cool the skin around the eyes.

Chapter Four: Skincare Products

Do you ever feel overwhelmed by the sheer number of skincare product companies out there? I know I do, and I'm in the business of skincare! There are choices at department stores, drug stores, spas, health food stores, farmers' markets, online, and through your friend or neighbor selling multi-level marketing products.

With so many choices, it is difficult to choose a product line that is safe, effective, and doesn't cost an arm and a leg. In keeping with our challenge to minimize the number of products, finding active-ingredient-rich products which allow us to use less, along with companies that don't push an extraordinary number of products (or come out with a new miracle elixir every month), is critical.

Let me make one thing clear that will help to greatly simplify your product choices: large, corporate skincare companies are not your friend.

A few reasons why:

o They are solely in business to make as much money as possible. They do this by using cheap, often toxic ingredients, marking up their products on average 80 percent, and selling you the largest quantity of products that they can. Most of these companies will spend huge amounts on advertising rather than improving their products.

o They use deceptive green- and natural-washing jargon to make you *think* their product is "green" or "natural," when the amount of these ingredients included is miniscule.

o There is virtually no oversight or regulations in the cosmetic industry. Remember, FDA stands for "Food and Drug

Administration," and they have very little jurisdiction over skincare companies.

o   Unless a large company is completely transparent in listing all their products' ingredients, you have no idea exactly what is in them (again, virtually no regulations in place here).

The best way to weed your way through this maze is to learn how to make an informed, educated choice.

The good news is, you have already accomplished one-half of this process by discovering the best ingredients for your skin type or condition, and the top ingredients for a specific result (exfoliate, moisturize, etc.). The second half is learning how to read a product label or ingredient list.

Unfortunately, this is not as easy as reading food labels, which are highly regulated and consistent. However, the following tips will help you understand the industry's labeling tricks and how to discern a quality skin or cosmetic product based on its label.

Reading a Skincare Product Label

Here are some considerations when reviewing skincare product labels or ingredient lists:

o   First of all, know there may not be a list of ingredients to read. Cosmetic companies do not have to list ingredients (yes, really!). Or they may just list *active* ingredients, but you have no way of knowing their concentration.

o   One regulation the FDA does require of health and beauty products is that their ingredients be listed using their International Nomenclature Cosmetic Ingredient (INCI) names, except for fragrances. This is to ensure consistency in labeling, yet it leads to more confusion because INCI names can be long and synthetic-sounding. In the ingredient section of this book, I have included the INCI names, when it is different than the common name, in parentheses. Note that on skincare products, the listing practice is the exact opposite—the INCI name is listed first and the common name is listed in parentheses, if the company lists the common name at all.

o Companies can list any ingredient in a concentration of less than 1 percent, in any order they choose. So that fantastic active ingredient can be listed first, yet have the lowest concentration of any ingredient in the product.

o Companies can "bundle" a group of ingredients under one ingredient name and only list that one ingredient on the label. They do this to hide toxin-producing ingredients when the public has become savvy to their potential harmful effects.

o Consumers are understandably concerned about toxic ingredients, and toxic preservatives have gained public attention lately. One manner of hiding a toxic preservative is the ability to list it simply as "fragrance," if the preservative has a scent.

So, what's a concerned consumer to do? Here are some tips to navigate skincare product labeling:

o Find a company that lists all ingredients (these lists may be on their website) and is completely transparent. Question if there is no ingredient list, or if the company chooses to list only active ingredients.

o Ingredients are listed in order of concentration, starting with the largest amount listed first (with the exception of those ingredients in concentrations of less than 1 percent). To keep it simple, look at just the first five ingredients and the last five ingredients. The first five are the core ingredients—this is where you should see some active ingredients. The last five will tell you how many fragrances, perfumes, colors, and preservatives are contained in the product. If all five ingredients listed last are in these categories, the product is probably overly fragranced, colored and/or preserved.

o   Usually, a short ingredient list is better than a long one.

Now let's talk about preservatives—another important skincare label topic. All products that contain water, or a water-derived ingredient such as hydrosol, require a preservative to guard against harmful bacteria, mold, and yeasts. Even if you make a homemade product containing water and keep it in the refrigerator, it will remain microbe-free for only a short period of time unless you include a preservative.

Many common cosmetic preservatives have been shown to be hormone disruptors or to release formaldehyde into the body. Parabens have gotten significant negative press lately on their toxicity.[19] There are healthier alternatives to look for, as listed below.

Note: some of these preservatives will be paired with others on the label to enhance their effectiveness and product shelf life, and their INCI name(s) appear in parentheses.

- Optiphen (phenoxyethanol, caprylyl glycol)
- Optiphen Plus (as above, and add sorbic acid)
- Cosmocil CQ (polyaminopropyl biguanide)
- Geogard (benzyl alcohol, dehydroacetic)
- Leucidal (lactobacillus ferment)
- Potassium Sorbate
- AM Ticide Coconut (lactobacillus and cocos nucifera fruit extract)

There are other completely natural (not just *derived* from nature) preservatives; however, if you see these on a product label, they will most likely be paired with a more full-spectrum preservative; or if not, they will require refrigeration and only last a few months. Some examples of completely natural preservatives are:

- Salicylic Acid
- Tea Tree Oil
- Grapefruit Seed Extract
- Thyme Essential Oil
- Bitter Orange Extract

If your favorite skincare product includes preservatives other than the ones listed here, research them to uncover any possible negative side effects. Also, make sure the concentration level of the preservatives is less than 1 percent. If it is higher, the product was formulated for a very long shelf life— good for retail stores, but not your face and health.

If you are looking for a new skincare product line, the best advice I can give you is to look for "small- batch, non-corporate" companies for four big reasons:

1. Typically, the people running these companies care more about your skin and making safe, natural products than their bottom line.
2. They don't have shareholders to answer to as to why their profit is not a million percent over cost.
3. They don't have to produce a product that will last some zillion years on the shelf or survive a long, hot trip on a truck for distribution.
4. And they don't have an astronomically-sized advertising budget. And because of these points, they usually produce a superior product.

You will find many of these companies through local advertising and online, but they can also be found in farmers' markets and boutique stores. To ensure quality control with these smaller businesses, make sure they have a professional and thorough website, as well as an easy way to contact them for questions or comments.

Buying products from a reputable spa is also a good bet. Although the skincare line may be expensive, it will contain high levels of active ingredients. These companies are usually the ones that have done, or utilize, the latest skin health research to create their skincare formulas. Spa skincare lines are larger than the small-batch companies I described above, but for the most part, they are small enough to produce a quality product without overusing preservatives.

The only drawback (besides the price) is that these products may be laden with fragrances which add to the "spa experience." Keep this in mind if you have any skin conditions, have sensitive skin, or want a "clean" (meaning no additives) skincare routine. You can also look for brands that contain 100 percent essential oils, botanicals, herbs, or are "fragrance-free."

Components of a Skincare Product

To better understand what is in our skincare products, let's disassemble one. All the following types of ingredients may be in a product:

Water: Just about every product contains water as its largest component. Our skin *needs* water (our skin consists of 70 percent water), so it is not awful to see this as the first ingredient listed. However, water brings down the cost of the product. Products that are formulated with other primary ingredients, such as aloe vera juice, will contain more nutrients and beneficial properties, but they will be more expensive.

Emulsifiers: Products need these to bind water to oil which creates a creamy consistency. Therefore, any product that contains both water (or an ingredient that contains water) and an oil, butter, or wax will contain an emulsifier.

Surfactants: These are the oil and dirt busters. They act by dissolving the oil and carrying the dirt away when rinsed off. You will find these in cleansers. Soap is a type of surfactant.

Liposomes: These are microscopic delivery systems. They "carry" other ingredients into deeper layers of the skin, which, it is believed, makes the ingredients more effective.

Fragrances, perfumes, and colors: Make the product look and smell nice.

Preservatives: Needed in any product that contains water or an ingredient with water.

Active Ingredients: These are all the ingredients that cause a beneficial change in your skin and are listed in Chapters Two and Three: exfoliators, antioxidants, hydrators (humectants), emollients, essential oils, peptides, plant stem cells, and hydrosols. In addition, botanicals, herbs, and other vitamins can also provide nourishment and positive effects to the skin.

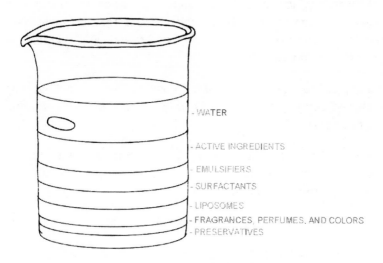

- WATER

- ACTIVE INGREDIENTS

- EMULSIFIERS

- SURFACTANTS

- LIPOSOMES

- FRAGRANCES, PERFUMES, AND COLORS

- PRESERVATIVES

Types of Products

Cleansers

Facial cleansers should be a no-brainer, right? After all, their purpose is simple: to clean your face. But choosing the right one for your skin type—one that's not too drying, too hydrating, too aggressive, or too mild—is another matter. To help you find the ideal cleanser for your skin, we need to dive into a short chemistry lesson again—but I promise to keep it short, educational, and fascinating.

However, before we do, some background information is important. There are two different types of cleansers: those with surfactants and those without. Surfactants, as mentioned above, are cleansing agents. Some types are also responsible for a foaming action when water is added. They fall into the categories of either soap or detergents. Soap is made from the combination of a plant oil or

96

animal fat mixed with an alkaline substance (usually sodium hydroxide or lye). When these are mixed, two byproducts are made: glycerin (a hydrator) and soap. Detergents are made synthetically. And, though it may seem counterintuitive, there is a type of detergent that is gentler on the skin than soap!

The reason relates to the pH (measure of acidity or alkalinity) of our skin. Our skin is acidic; it lands around 5.5 on the pH scale. Products of similar pH to our skin will not strip the acid mantle of naturally-produced oils and will help to keep our skin flora in balance. What we need to look for in a cleanser is a more *acidic* pH. Soap runs between 9.0 and 10.5—way too alkaline for our skin. The one exception is glycerin soap (also spelled glycerine), where the byproduct, glycerin, is left in the soap mixture. Soaps that include oils, such as coconut and olive, will be closer in pH to our skin, but are probably still too alkaline to keep facial skin healthy—though they are fine for the body, especially if you apply lotion, body butter, or body cream after cleansing.

Note: lots of people love Castile soap—but it is not ideal for facial cleansing as it has a pH of 8.9.

pH CHART

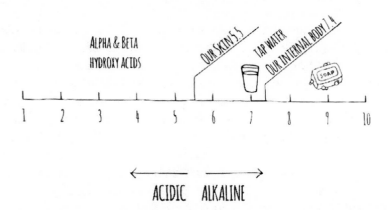

ALPHA & BETA
HYDROXY ACIDS

OUR SKIN 5.5

TAP WATER

OUR INTERNAL BODY 7.4

SOAP

1   2   3   4   5   6   7   8   9   10

←——————   ——————→
ACIDIC   ALKALINE

Mild surfactants (like those listed below) are closest to our skin's pH and the least likely cleansing agent to irritate the skin. The gentlest surfactants are called "non-ionic." It is important to note that products with non-ionic surfactants will not lather or foam; however, they are still cleansing the skin.

Some of the best surfactants to look for on an ingredient list are:

- CocoBetaine
- Decyl Polyglucoside
- Decyl Glucoside
- Lauryl Glucoside
- Polysorbatepoly 20
- Polysorbate 80
- PEG-60 Almond Glycerides
- Glyceryl Cocoate
- Sucrose Cocoate

Harsher, and less healthy, surfactants to stay away from are:

- Sodium Lauryl (or Laureth) Sulfate (the most common and the worst!)
- Ammonium Lauryl (or Laureth) Sulfate
- Stearic Acid
- Lauric Acid
- Myristic Acid
- palmiti
- Palmitic Acid

Why don't all skincare products list their pH levels? It would be helpful, yet you will hardly ever find this description on a commercial product. However, quality products will be fairly in-line with the skin's pH level, because if they weren't, they would harm the skin with dryness and inflammation, and no one would buy them. The exceptions are treatment-focused products, such as AHAs. These will be more acidic to better exfoliate and attain desired results. If you have sensitive skin or rosacea, it is imperative you choose products that are mild and gentle, specifically formulated to align with the skin's pH. If you have acne, don't fall prey to products that are too harsh for the sake of drying out your existing blemishes. These products are usually exceptionally *alkaline*, and they will disrupt skin flora, causing the skin to be more susceptible to the acne bacteria, *P. acnes*, which will cause more breakouts in the long run.

Of course, there is another way to clean your skin properly: use products that don't contain surfactants at all. These cleansers take the form of a cleansing cream, cleansing milk, or facial oil. They usually include fruit acids, honey, and oils. These mildly cleansing ingredients, coupled with the rubbing action of your fingertips, will clean the skin.

Just keep in mind that if you wear makeup, have very oily skin, or come into a great deal of dirt or air pollution during the day, these non-surfactant cleansers may not do the trick. However, for your morning cleanse or on no-makeup days, they are amazing for all skin types—especially dry, mature, or sensitive skin.

You can also "make" an effective cleanser from items found in your kitchen. I have a friend who only uses coconut milk to wash her face. Or an oil cleanser (there are many on the market these days) made from an oil or combination of skin-nourishing oils is excellent. To make your own cleanser: find a single oil recommended for your type of skin in the skincare ingredients section of this book, or try some of the "Do-It-Yourself" oil-blend cleansers recommended below:

<u>DIY Oil-Blend Cleansers</u>

- ❖ Dry Skin: olive, avocado, and fractionated coconut oil
- ❖ Normal/Combo Skin: olive, rice bran, and hazelnut oil
- ❖ Oily Skin: grapeseed, hazelnut, and evening primrose oil (may need to apply a mild surfactant cleanser on top of the oil)
- ❖ Blemish-prone Skin: grapeseed, hemp seed, and neem oil (may need to apply a mild surfactant cleanser on top of the oil)
- ❖ Sensitive Skin: rice bran, calendula, and hemp seed oil

Mix these combinations in equal amounts. Keep in a small, dark-colored glass container. Larger mixtures should be kept in the refrigerator.

If you have oily and/or blemish-prone skin, you may be reluctant to wash with oil exclusively. I have oily skin, which is at times blemish-prone, and what I have done in the past is mix half a dispenser bottle with a mild surfactant cleanser and the other half with grapeseed oil. If you use this formula, just remember to shake the bottle before each use. With this method, you get the nutrients and skin conditioning benefits of the oil along with the cleansing properties of the cleanser.

A note about cleansing your skin with water exclusively: I know women who do this, and it is the ultimate in simple skincare—but I don't recommend it. All tap water is chemically treated to be highly alkaline to prevent city water pipes from rusting (if you have access to well water, this information may not apply depending upon the pH of your well water). Therefore, city tap water is not in alignment with our skin's pH level. One caveat: if you follow a water cleanse with a product that contains oil, it will better neutralize the alkalinity in the water. Apply while your skin is damp, and it will lock in the hydrating effect of the water.

Should you scrub your face clean? Cleansing grains or facial brushes are very popular, and I admit that my face does feel so much cleaner and smoother after I use one. Using these devices or scrubs are a form of manual exfoliation, and exfoliating your skin is key to keeping your skin fresh and healthy. However, I have found in my work that most people use these devices or scrubs way too often (enter that great feeling after you use them). If you like the idea of an electronic brush, make sure it *vibrates* rather than *rotates*, and use with a "sensitive" brush head. I do not recommend grainy scrubs at all unless they are made with gentler beeswax, castor, or jojoba wax beads. Thicker, more resilient skin can get away with manual exfoliation twice a week, normal skin only once a week. If you have mature and/or sensitive skin, stick to chemical exfoliation. In addition, if you have acne or any blemishes, NEVER use manual exfoliation. The harmful bacteria that are in most blemishes will spread to other pores and cause more breakouts.

Toners

Toners play a variety of roles for your skin—from removing any traces of cleanser or remaining dirt and makeup after you wash your face, to preparing your skin for any serums or treatments. They also replenish and rebalance the acid mantle, and may contain beneficial antioxidants, soothing agents, or hydrating ingredients. If your skin is not overly oily or blemished, toners can be used in place of a cleanser in the morning (lately advertised in the form of "micellar cleansing water", which is simply a type of toner). I use a toner after I work out to lightly clean the skin and remove sweat, which can attract dirt.

Although toners do have benefits, they are not essential in a skincare routine. Before you invest in a toner, consider how it will add to your skincare routine. For example, do you have extra dry skin that would benefit from a toner containing hydrating hyaluronic acid and rose? Or, if you have *slightly dry skin,* could a toner serve as your hydrating product? Could your occasional blemishes be remedied with a toner containing salicylic acid (willow bark) and neem extract? Do you have sensitive skin that would benefit from a toner containing aloe vera juice and green tea extract, allowing this product to replace a serum with similar ingredients? The point is, to keep things simple, be discriminating before automatically including a toner in your skincare routine.

Another option is to make your own toner by purchasing **essential oil hydrosols** based on the properties you desire. For hydrosol-based toners, make sure to separate a small amount to keep with your skincare supplies, and plan to store the rest in the refrigerator, as hydrosols do go bad. Here is a great toner blend for acne/blemish-prone skin, that includes apple cider vinegar and aloe vera:

DIY Acne/Blemish-Prone Toner

- ❖ 1 part Apple Cider Vinegar
- ❖ 3 parts Tea Tree Hydrosol
- ❖ 1 part Lavender Hydrosol
- ❖ 1 part Aloe Vera Juice

Shake before use and keep refrigerated.

Serums and Treatments

Serums are skincare powerhouses. They contain the greatest amount of active ingredients, proportionately, to treat or affect change in your skin. Serums are used for three purposes:

- o   To focus on a specific skin goal
- o   To intensify the strength of a skincare routine
- o   To round out the ingredients in a regime for a more comprehensive practice

Typically, you will find distinct serums that act as one of the following:

- o   A hydrator (see section later in this chapter for more information on hydrating serums)
- o   An antioxidant
- o   A pigment control and brightening agent
- o   A healing and soothing agent (many times listed as "anti-redness")
- o   An "anti-aging" serum for mature skin (or I came across one called "wrinkle-release")

To determine recommended active ingredients most effective for your type of skin or to address a   particular condition, review the ingredients listed in *Chapter Three: Skin Types and Conditions, and the   Skincare Ingredients Best for Each.*

There are also combination serums on the market, such as one I found named a "rejuvenating serum," which includes antioxidants and calming agents. If you can't decide on your highest priority skincare   concern, you may wish to look for an all-in-one serum. Serums can also include various vitamins,   botanicals, and herbs.

The key to serums is knowing how and when to use them. **The adage, "protect during the day, and help   repair during the night," is**

important to remember. For example, antioxidants boost your sunscreen's protective ability while providing other benefits, such as improving skin tone. Therefore, it's best to apply an antioxidant serum in the morning before your sunscreen (however, it can be applied both day and evening). A hydrating serum should be applied at night before your moisturizer or facial oil (unless you have extremely dry skin, then use it day and night). Other serums are used in the morning, at night, or both, depending on your needs.

Note: only the smallest amount of serum is needed. I won't say "just a drop," because sometimes it takes more than that to cover your face, but do use the least amount possible. If it feels like you have applied a mask, you have used too much.

When a product specifically addresses acne or retinoic exfoliation, it is called a *treatment*. The best acne treatments contain salicylic acid (BHA) and/or tea tree oil. They may also contain calming agents, such as aloe vera and green tea extract, to soothe irritation that comes with a breakout. It is best to start slowly with an acne treatment that contains salicylic acid so that you don't over-dry your skin. In the beginning, apply at night and eventually add a morning application, if needed.

Retinol treatments should only be applied at night because they cause photo-sensitivity to the sun. Once you apply a retinol treatment, wait a few minutes to let the retinol absorb (I brush my teeth during this time) before applying other products. It is wise to read the label on retinol products, as many contain hydrators, enabling you to forgo a hydrating serum. However, like salicylic acid products, retinol can be drying, so start out with a product that contains a small concentration and increase from there.

Boosters

Booster products, mostly found in serums, are meant to enhance the amount of active ingredients in a product. For example, if you apply a hydrating serum containing hyaluronic acid, a booster will contain a super-concentrated amount of hyaluronic acid to be applied on top of the serum. Personally, I don't see the value in boosters. If you want to boost your serum, why not just apply another layer? I believe it is another tactic skincare companies use to increase the number of products we buy. In my mind, it's a total rip-off.

Hydrating Serums and Moisturizers

Sometimes the terms "hydrators" and "moisturizers" are used interchangeably, yet they perform very different functions.

As stated before, hydrators absorb water from the air and bind it to the skin. They are good for dehydrated skin which lacks water. A hydrating serum can also be multifunctional by containing beneficial botanicals or oil. A moisturizer's main function is to prevent transepidermal water loss (TEWL) by forming a barrier over the skin. They retain the moisture that is already present on the skin when applied by creating a protective seal, or what is also known as an "occlusive effect." This seal helps keep skin cells healthy so that they produce an appropriate amount of oil, as well as coating the skin with a light layer of oil to aid the acid mantle.

Moisturizers are known to be good for dry skin; however, you can probably see how well hydrators and moisturizers work together. Hydrating serums attract water to the skin, and moisturizers seal the water in and leave a protective barrier that prevents further water loss.

So, in a simple beauty routine, do you need both a moisturizer and a hydrator?

In many cases, no. Remember, your acid mantle already contains water and oil, so the mechanism to hydrate and moisturize our skin is in place. These products should come into play only if you feel your skin needs further assistance. Specifically, if you have dry skin—especially if you have both premature aging and dry skin—it is a super advantageous to use both.

There are also multitasking moisturizers that contain hydrating ingredients; therefore, you only need to purchase one product that performs both functions. Just keep in mind, if you have very dry skin, a combo moisturizer may not be as effective as using a separate serum under a moisturizer. If you have premature aging skin that is not dry, you can try a hydrating serum that includes a small amount of oil (which many do) and skip the moisturizer. This also applies to those who do not have dry skin but live in dry climates, or who are smokers. If you have oily skin with flaking, then your skin is probably dehydrated. Drink more water and apply a hydrating serum before bed (again, no need to use a separate moisturizer).

Pure oil, on its own, is a wonderful moisturizer. Surprisingly, since many do not add a greasy feel to the skin they are fine to apply in the morning. Some even have natural sunscreen capabilities, such as Rosehip Seed Oil, Sea Buckthorn Seed Oil, and Avocado Oil, adding to the benefit of morning application. Others are highly emollient and great for dry skin, but best applied at night. Every oil mentioned in this book, plus other non-synthetic oils, have nutritive skincare properties, including soothing, softening, restoring, and toning. They also have the moisturizing effects of protecting the skin by supporting the skin barrier, while allowing the skin to breathe.

DIY Premature Aging Skin Facial Oil Blend

- ❖ 3 parts Argan Oil
- ❖ 1 part Rosehip Seed Oil
- ❖ 1 part Cranberry Seed Oil

Keep in a small, dark-glass dropper bottle. Store excess oil blend in the refrigerator.

An Amazing Hydration Trick:

This is one of my favorite techniques for increasing hydration in the skin. And the best part is that any skin can benefit from it. After you cleanse your face, spray your face with an appropriate hydrosol or toner, and do not wipe it off. With your face moist from the hydrosol or toner, apply your next product: serum, sunscreen, moisturizer, or facial oil. The "moisture", as well as any other therapeutic ingredients from the hydrosol or toner, will be sealed into the skin by the next product applied. Even oily and acne/blemish-prone skin can become dehydrated, and the tea tree extract (found in tea tree hydrosol) or salicylic acid (found in many blemish-control toners) won't be wiped away by a cotton ball. Sensitive skin and rosacea benefit the most from helichrysum or chamomile hydrosol, and dry and premature aging skin do best with rose or frankincense hydrosol. For an all-around, skin-nourishing hydrator use geranium hydrosol.

Sunscreen

I'm often asked the question: What are the most essential skincare products? My top three:

1. Sunscreen
2. Sunscreen
3. Sunscreen

This gives you an idea of how essential it is to protect your skin from the sun's ultraviolet rays, or UV rays.

Our big, beautiful sun is also the biggest toxin-producer to our skin. Though some sunlight is beneficial, it can also cause a myriad of problems including sun spots, wrinkles, sagging skin and, worst of all, cancer.

Pigmentation to the skin happens when melanocytes are exposed to UV rays, causing them to produce a dark substance called melanin. Because this darker color absorbs more sun rays, it acts as a natural sun protection when it is absorbed into surrounding skin cells. These darkened cells rise to the top of the epidermis and create a temporary tan. A tan signals sun damage. Hyperpigmentation is a condition whereby the darkened cells remain as permanent sun spots, which are very difficult to remove. People of color can also get sun damage, although there is less actual darkening because their darker complexions protect them more from the sun than lighter complexions.

UV rays also damage the elastin skin fibers and increase the number of those pesky free radicals, leading to wrinkling and sagging of the skin. When harm to DNA occurs from UV exposure, skin cancer can develop. The sun also provides the benefit of vitamin D production, but keep in mind that a small amount of exposure can generate sufficient amounts.[20]

Sunscreen ingredients protect against the sun's UV rays. There are two types of UV rays: UVB and UVA. UVB rays are responsible for turning the skin red or tan, causing damage to the skin. UVA rays also cause harm, but in the form of wrinkles. SPF—or sun protection factor—is the measurement of time it takes the skin to turn red when exposed to the sun; thus, it only applies to UVB rays. However, if a label uses the wording **Broad Spectrum**, it must shield against UVA rays proportional to the SPF value.[21] Therefore, **you should always look for labels that indicate this complete protection.** Sunscreen ingredients are classified as either a chemical or physical-based (also called mineral sunscreen).

Chemical ingredients absorb the sun rays, and most are highly toxic. The physical ingredients, **titanium dioxide** and **zinc oxide**, reflect and scatter UV rays, and because they rest on top of the skin and are not absorbed, they are considered non-toxic. Although titanium dioxide is commonly included in this group, zinc oxide is the only sunscreen ingredient approved by the FDA to effectively protect against both UVA and UVB rays.[22] If that's not enough to get you to look for zinc oxide in your sunscreen, it is also known to help heal wounds, aid in the recovery of burns and damaged tissue, improve synthesis of collagen, lower inflammation, and treat both acne and rosacea. Talk about a multitasker!

SPF factors, the numbers listed after "SPF" on the packaging, are not as important as they seem. The key is to choose a product with at least 15 SPF factor. As the number rises beyond 15, the actual increase in protection does not increase proportionately. SPF 30 has only four percent greater protection than SPF 15. A better way to protect your skin is to reapply sunscreen throughout the day, rather than choosing a higher SPF. If you wear makeup, find one that includes SPF factor, and try powders that include sun protection for easy reapplication throughout the day. And always remember to apply every day—including cloudy and rainy days, as UVA rays are still abundant during this time.

Sunscreen is the only product listed in this book that you may not find in "small-batch, non-corporate" skincare companies. The reason for this is that testing, and the process for applying for and receiving the government approval to display an SPF designation, is very expensive. Nevertheless, there are many high-quality sunscreens on the market. Sunscreen products sold in spas are one choice, and the Environmental Working Group (www.ewg.org) publishes a very comprehensive guide to sunscreens. You can sign up for updates from EWG via their newsletter.

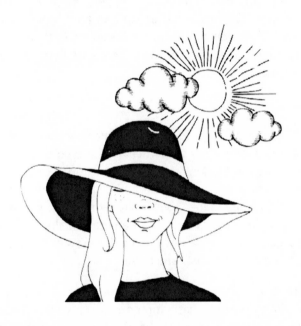

So, apply that sunscreen! It is much easier to prevent sun damage than it is to repair it.

Eye Products

Eye creams and gels are typically soothing hydrators and moisturizers that are safe to use around the eye. They are not absolutely *needed* in a skincare routine, but many people love them to address puffiness, dark circles, or reduce the appearance of crow's feet. In addition, the skin in the area around the eyes does not have as many oil glands as the rest of your face, so an extra boost of hydration and moisturization from an eye treatment will help with dryness and crepeyness. In the past, I was an eye cream aficionado, thinking they were more emollient than gels. However, some of the newer eye gels are very moisturizing and have wonderful cooling effects. Also, they seem to sink into the skin faster than creams. It is personal preference which one you choose—or if you choose to use them at all, based on your skin.

Masks

Masks are specialty skincare products, usually applied once a week. In most cases, masks treat a particular skin type or condition. For example, masks for dry skin hydrate and moisturize, and can include ingredients such as hyaluronic acid and collagen. If your skin is red and inflamed, a mask made specifically for sensitive skin will soothe and calm, with ingredients such as green tea and aloe vera. Oily and congested skin should use a mask that helps draw out impurities with ingredients such as charcoal and clay.

Masks are also a good exfoliation method for all skin types. For example, an exfoliating mask for normal, dry, or oily skin may contain BHA (salicylic acid/willow bark), AHAs, and/or fruit enzymes. Exfoliating masks for sensitive skin or rosacea should only include mandelic acid, azelaic acid, and/or papaya (papain) enzyme. People with skin conditions, such as dermatitis, eczema, and psoriasis, should only use a mask that contains papaya (papain) as an exfoliating agent.

Mask Tips:

o A mask should be applied after you cleanse (and tone, if you use toner), but before any serums or moisturizers are put on.
o Use a good amount—this is where you can go a bit overboard—and wait 10 to 20 minutes before removing.
o Wash off the mask with water only or using a soft washcloth and warm water. Or if the mask is creamy and for dry skin, wipe off the excess with a tissue or cotton round, but leave some on to work overnight.

There are many masks that you can make yourself:

❖ For dry skin: mash up an avocado.
❖ To zap blemishes: mix charcoal powder or Matcha green tea powder with tea tree hydrosol.
❖ To soothe and purify sensitive skin: combine rose, sea, or kaolin clay with aloe vera juice. Add a few drops of helichrysum essential oil to boost the therapeutic effect.
❖ For all skin types: simply massage aloe vera gel into the skin and let dry.

<u>DIY Exfoliating Mask</u>

❖ 4 chunks of pineapple
❖ ½ ripe papaya
❖ 1 tablespoon of local honey

Mix pineapple and papaya together in blender. Check consistency and add a teaspoon of water if   needed. Add honey and blend.

Oily and thicker skins can leave on 20 minutes. Sensitive and mature skin, leave on no more than 10   minutes. If the tingling turns into a burning sensation, remove mask with warm water and a soft wash cloth.

Sensitive skin, as well as skin with dermatitis, eczema, or psoriasis, can substitute aloe vera gel instead of the pineapple for a therapeutic treatment mask.

DIY Probiotic Skin Balancing Mask

- ❖ A mashed avocado or aloe vera gel (Avocado if you have dry skin—including dry *and* sensitive skin. Aloe vera gel if you have oily skin—including oily *and* sensitive skin. If your skin falls in between dry and oily, use both.)
- ❖ 1 probiotic capsule (see *Chapter Six: Skin Nutrition* for how to choose an effective probiotic supplement), opened, discard capsule coating

Mix all ingredients well. Apply and leave on face for approximately 15 minutes. Remove with warm water.

The Best Treatment for Blackheads and Large Pores

Blackheads and large pores are the bane of so many women! These are the most common concerns I hear when consulting with my esthetician clients. They tend to be an issue with people with skin that leans on the oily side, but they can affect all skin types. First of all, pores can only be minimized temporarily by applying an astringent- type product (but don't get confused and use a product named an astringent that contains alcohol). Find suggestions for these products in the oily skin ingredient section of this book. Blackheads are not dirt that has been trapped in your pores, but naturally-produced oil that darkens when exposed to oxygen, which will harden if not removed. Larger pores allow this oil to pool, and, therefore, the oxygenation is more visible. One commercial solution is nose strips. They work by pulling the darkened and hardened oil out of the pores. These strips only work if the oil has been allowed to harden in the pores. I have experienced better success with the following treatment:

1. Gently steam your face (optional, but optimal).
2. Wash your face with warm water and an enzyme cleanser.
3. Apply a charcoal, clay, or moor mud mask on your nose and the cheek area around your nose. (The most aggressive masks are French green clay and moor mud.) Leave on skin for 10 minutes, then rinse off with warm water and a wash cloth.
4. Apply an AHA and salicylic acid serum.
5. If you have normal to dry skin apply a thin coating of grapeseed oil or jojoba oil. If you have oily or acne/blemish-prone skin, skip this step.

Apply no more than once a week. Not recommended if you have sensitive skin or rosacea.

Chapter Five: Spa Treatments and DIY Facials

Treat yourself to a facial—yes, really!

You may be thinking: how can getting facials fit into a simplified skincare routine? I know it sounds crazy, but hear me out. With our streamlined skincare concept, we want to minimize the number of products we use daily and save time with a shortened skincare regime. But, we also want to maintain, or even surpass, the glowy and healthy results.

We, in the United States, think of facials as a luxury. But many cultures consider facials preventative maintenance, just like we think of dental teeth cleaning here. The French have always placed a greater focus on skin health, rather than on cosmetics, to highlight beauty. And Koreans make it a family outing to go to a spa for treatments. **Even though it is valuable to consider the relaxation and pampering aspect of facials, especially in our high-stress society, emphasis should also be placed on facials' aim of improving the health of our skin.**

It's already been established that regular exfoliation is highly beneficial and for all skin types since it removes the top layer of dull, dead skin cells, revs up the skin regeneration process, and allows active ingredients applied after an exfoliation to penetrate deeper into the skin layers. So, I'm suggesting that instead of a daily or weekly exfoliation product, most skin types will benefit just as much, if not more, from a monthly facial that includes a deep exfoliation. (For mature skin, or for those looking to delay the effects of aging as much as possible, I recommend applying a retinol treatment nightly, even if you are receiving a monthly facial.) Other benefits to a

119

regular facial are improving skin tone and texture; stimulating the production of collagen and elastin; increasing moisture retention; and creating a rosy, healthy glow.

Another perk of a professional facial is that **your skin will be getting a dose of therapeutic skin ingredients typically not contained in home-care products.** In addition, since stress plays a big role in skin problems, spending an hour a month pampering yourself will soothe your soul just as much as your skin. If you are worried about cost, try a beauty or skincare school where senior students perform the facials at a much lower price than spas. A school facial may not include serums, and probably won't include any specialized treatments, but all essential components will be offered.

A typical facial will include:

1. Cleansing the face
2. Applying toner
3. Exfoliation, typically with fruit enzymes and/or AHAs
4. Facial massage with oil (sometimes a shoulder, head, and arm massage is included) **A facial massage is very beneficial, helping your lymph and blood supply to oxygenate your skin and remove toxins more efficiently, as well as helping to relax tight muscles while brightening your face with a healthy glow.**
5. Extractions, if needed (may not be done at a school)
6. Mask application
7. Serum(s) application (may not be used at a school)
8. Moisturizer application (Sunscreen could be included in the moisturizer or applied separately.)
9. Eye treatment application
10. Lip treatment application

In a spa, each step will be individualized based on your skin type, condition, and your goals. In a school, you may receive a more generic facial, but you will still walk out feeling an improvement in your skin. Since there are many "add-ons" available with a facial, a visit to a spa can wind up being a not-so-simple endeavor. Just like with skincare products, don't feel like you *need* to boost your facial. Although add-on   services can be valuable, know that you are not missing out if you don't include them.

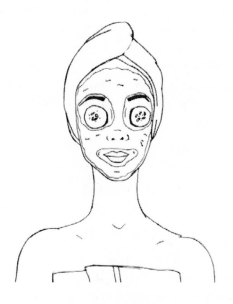

There is one additional service I want to talk about because it is often misunderstood, and that is a facial peel. Ten years ago, peels were something you received in a dermatologist's or plastic surgeon's office, and you walked out looking like your skin had melted off your face—red and raw. These peels still exist, and they are one option if you have deep acne or other scars; however, the peels offered today run a whole range from very superficial to deeper into the epidermis. In fact, a typical facial could be called a "peel," because the top layer of dead skin cells is removed during the exfoliation step.

As you may recall from Chapter One, the epidermis has five layers of skin and the top layer is called the stratum corneum. The stratum corneum is made up of fifteen to twenty layers of dead skin cells.

Therefore, spa peels can remove one to twenty layers of cells depending on their strength. Stronger peels can go even further and penetrate layers below the stratum corneum to deeper layers within the epidermis, causing visual peeling that begins approximately two to three days after the peel. But, spa peels will go no deeper than the epidermis. To peel down to the dermis requires a physician's directive and supervision. **With superficial peels, you may not experience any visible skin peeling at all, but your skin will still gain all the benefits.**

The benefits of a peel are:

- o Improves skin texture, including smoothing scars
- o Reduces the effects of sun damage, including hyperpigmentation
- o Improves skin tone
- o Increases moisture retention
- o Improves skin barrier function
- o Stimulates the production of collagen and elastin

Choose a type of peel based on your goals. If you have age spots, sun spots, scarring, or very rough, dull skin, a deeper peel would be best. These are done about every six months to once a year; just keep in mind that you may receive comments on the appearance of your skin (as it will start peeling) if you go out in public during the visible peeling stage. When I received a deep peel, I took a Friday off work (which was 3 days after the peel when the most peeling began for me) and stayed at home the following weekend and caught up on all the books I had wanted to read for ages. Also, keep in mind that if you get a face peel and a décolleté peel simultaneously, the different areas may not peel at the same rate— your face or chest may peel faster than the other.

For a gentler option, you can receive a more superficial peel once a month with no down time. You will still reap all the benefits listed above, but to a lesser degree than with a deeper peel. Some estheticians recommend a peel twice a month for treating acne. For more specific recommendations, talk to an esthetician about her suggestions.

Another little-known service available with a facial or a peel is a skin analysis. Before any facial-type   service, an esthetician will ask you several questions and study your skin under a magnifying glass to determine the best combination of products for the facial to meet your skincare goals. The information   gathered is then used to recommend a home-care regimen. Your esthetician will probably suggest products sold by her spa, but do not feel pressured to buy these products if you don't want to. I promise, you will not hurt her feelings. Most estheticians want to share their expert knowledge and are simply happy that their client is pleased with their work. Bring the tear-out sheets from this book, or make notes in your phone or on a notepad. When booking your appointment, ask if the visit includes a consultation before the service. If it doesn't, you can probably book one before the actual facial or peel, free of charge. Most skincare schools offer a consultation before a facial as part of their curriculum.

If spa treatments just aren't your thing, a monthly home facial is your best bet. These are great if you are able to tune out everything else that is going on in your home, relax, and enjoy the experience.

Another fun idea is to make a monthly "date" with a friend (or friends) for a spa night—kind of like a grown-up slumber party that also gives you the excuse to catch up over a few glasses of wine. The only drawback to a home facial is the need to purchase more products. However, this purchase will last several months and may be simpler than driving to a spa or beauty school each month.

Recipe for a Home Facial

Prep: Have all products set out and ready to use. Dampen two hand towels, fold them length-wise (hotdog style), and roll them both up. Place one on a microwave-safe plate or bowl for heating, and leave one at room temperature.

1. Rub a few drops of balancing or soothing essential oil (lavender is very common) between your palms, and hold your hands about 5 inches away from your nose. Take at least three deep breaths with your inhale, filling your belly. Or, if you have an essential oil diffuser, this is a good time to use it—but still do the deep breathing.
2. Wash your face and remove all makeup.
3. Apply toner or hydrosol.
4. Apply a fruit enzyme product, or blend half a ripe papaya with a few chunks of pineapple and apply to your face. *If you have sensitive skin or a skin condition, omit the pineapple chunks and only use a mashed papaya.*
5. Warm the first damp towel in the microwave for 30-40 seconds (make sure the towel is not too hot, though it should be nice and warm), and, while lying down with the fruit enzyme product or blended fruit still on your face, wrap your face with the towel. The heat from the towel will open the pores and allow the enzymes to work better. Relax for 10 minutes or shorten the time if tingling from the mask becomes a burning sensation.
6. Remove fruit enzymes with the damp towel.

7. Apply toner or hydrosol (optional). If you use only a clay mask in the next step, you may want to wait to apply toner until after the mask to ensure all product is removed.

8. Apply a clay, AHA/BHA, or hydrating mask depending on your skin type. Relax with the mask on for 15 minutes. Remove with the second room-temperature damp towel. Or, for a super- charged facial, apply a clay or AHA/BHA mask, wait 10 minutes, and remove with damp towel. Then apply hydrating mask, wait another 10 minutes, and remove by rinsing with cool water. While your mask is on your face, this is a good time to repeat rubbing the essential oil on your palms and breathing deeply.

9. If you waited to apply the toner until after the mask, apply toner now.

10. Apply any preferred serums, or a retinol or salicylic acid treatment.

11. Apply moisturizer or facial oil. If you like, a few drops of essential oil recommended for your skin type or a skincare blend, can be added to the oil. Massage the moisturizer or oil in small circles in an upward direction on your face.

12. Apply eye cream or gel and lip balm.

13. If you have hydrosol in a spray container, lightly mist your face with it.

14. Relax and enjoy how fantastic your face feels!

Chapter Six: Skin Nutrition

You have probably heard the adage: don't eat chocolate if you want clear skin. And although many people can eat chocolate without experiencing skin problems, this old saying has some truth to it.

Our skin directly reflects the foods we eat. In fact, the condition of our skin mirrors what is happening in our gut. What we eat has a direct effect on skin conditions, such as acne and rosacea, and on our skin's ability to produce collagen and elastin, regenerate cells, and generally delay the signs of aging.

In her book, *Clean Skin from Within*, Dr. Trevor Cates lists six causes of unhealthy skin:[23]

1. Inflammation
2. Microbiome disturbance (both skin and intestinal flora)
3. Oxidative damage
4. Blood sugar issues
5. Nutritional deficiencies
6. Hormonal imbalances

Although the environment plays an enormous role in oxidative damage, nutrition is linked to all six causes. This is pretty depressing news if you are like me and enjoy the conveniences of all the food and meal choices today. The good news is that with a few changes, you can start seeing healthier skin. And along the way, you may start noticing better energy, sleep, and overall well-being, which will inspire you to make a few *more* healthy substitutions, leading to your best skin yet. Plus, if you make a commitment to clean up your diet, your skin may start looking so great that you require less skincare products.

Although my focus is normally on the positive actions we can take to improve our skin, let's delve into the dark side of these six skin wreckers to underscore why good nutrition is so important.

1. Inflammation—this can occur invisibly within our bodies, such as in digestive stress; or visibly, such as in a sprained ankle. Internal inflammation occurs whenever your body deems something as a threat, including food allergies or intolerances, toxins, and sometimes medications. If you suffer from a severe or unexplained skin condition, such as eczema, psoriasis, or even continual acne breakouts (ruling out hormonal causes), I suggest you see a health professional about receiving a food sensitivity test.

   For the rest of us, hidden inflammation can occur from eating a diet full of refined grains, sugar, fried foods, artificial sweeteners, partially-hydrogenated fat, packaged foods containing additives   and preservatives, and, in many cases, dairy. Eating an excess of these foods disturbs our intestinal microbiome, or flora, which causes the lining of our stomach and intestines to become permeable, allowing food particles to enter our blood stream. This condition is officially called "Leaky Gut Syndrome".

   The body sees these food bits as foreign invaders and creates inflammation in an attempt to fight them off. It is not exactly known how or why, but this constant inflammation shows up in various ways throughout the body including skin conditions, or in less severe cases, premature aging.

   The first step to combatting inflammation is to determine if you are sensitive or allergic to any   foods and eliminate them from your diet. The good news is, if you are merely *sensitive* as opposed to *allergic*, you may be able to reintroduce these foods at a later date. In addition, eat an anti-inflammatory diet that is high in fresh, organic fruits and vegetables; has moderate amounts of free-range meats, fish, seafood; and contains a small amount of primarily whole grains (1-2 servings per day).

2. Microbiome and flora—you've heard those terms before, right? Just like the skin has its own beneficial bacteria colony, so does the gut. And just like internal inflammation, if stomach and intestinal flora is disrupted leading to a preponderance of detrimental bacteria, it will not only cause intestinal problems, but could show up as skin conditions. Specifically, if you suffer from acne, an imbalanced gut microbiome could be one of the causes.

    To supply your body with good bacteria, eat fermented foods, such as sauerkraut or kimchi, or drink kombucha that is not too high in sugar. Some yogurt contains probiotic cultures, but make sure it is low in sugar; if you are sensitive to dairy look for a dairy substitute, such as coconut milk or cashew milk yogurt. You can also choose to take a **probiotic supplement. If you go this route, make sure it is a refrigerated brand and contains at least 25 billion CFUs and 7 strains of beneficial bacteria. Also, it is best to take probiotic supplements at night on an empty stomach.**

3. Oxidative damage—this comes from UV rays; or, oxidative damage can come from free radicals developed internally, which can lead to chronic diseases and premature aging. Free radicals are created internally from fried foods, charred foods (such as from barbequing), alcohol, and pesticides on produce. Other foods that cause free radicals to flourish are hydrogenated fats, highly processed foods, and rancid oil (buy oil in small, dark glass bottles and if it smells

bad, throw it out). To reduce these cell-bombing free radicals, cut back on the above listed foods and eat antioxidant-rich foods.

Foods high in antioxidants include:

- Berries (blueberries, blackberries, strawberries, raspberries, elderberries, and cranberries)
- Red and purple grapes
- Beans (white, kidney, pinto, red, and black)
- Nuts (almonds, pecans, walnuts, and hazelnuts)
- Apples
- And (hooray!) dark chocolate

4. Sugar—you've probably heard the horror stories about sugar, and unfortunately, especially where your skin is concerned, they are all true. Eating too much sugar can lead to a host of skin problems. One of the effects of consuming high-glycemic foods (sugar and foods that turn to sugar quickly in the body, such as refined grains) is an increase in glycation. Glycation is the process in which excess sugars connect to proteins, including collagen and elastin, producing Advanced Glycation End Products (AGEs). These end products create stiff, rigid bonds in the proteins, leading to wrinkles, thinning, sagging, and a reduced ability for the skin to repair itself.

Dull, dry complexions are also the result of AGEs. What's more, glycation causes inflammation, possibly sparking additional skin problems. Sugar and other high-glycemic foods also increase insulin in the bloodstream, which can cause an increase in sebum production, possibly triggering an acne breakout.

Consequently, the goal for all skin types is to slow glycation by reducing our sugar and refined grain intake. Regrettably, in our modern grocery store environment, this is not the easiest thing to do because sugar is added to almost all packaged products. **This does not make shopping simple, but if you are like me and don't want to cook everything from scratch, begin reading labels.**

Here are some tips to help you get started:

- o You can find salad dressing, nut butters, and pasta sauce without added sugar.
- o Regarding packaged grains, look for brown or sprouted grains.
- o Purchase only whole grain breads and crackers.
- o Beware of fruits that are high in sugar (such as most tropical fruits, including bananas), and only eat fruit with their skins, as the fiber included in the skin will slow down the absorption of sugar. And, as a bonus, the skins are loaded with nutrients.
- o This goes for potatoes too—eat the skin.
- o Strictly limit sugary drinks, including fruit juice. Don't add sugar to coffee, tea, or smoothies.
- o Substitute 100 percent pure stevia, a natural herbal sweetener, for sugar.
- o Also, sadly, alcohol turns almost immediately to sugar in our systems; so, enjoy in moderation, and avoid sweet alcoholic drinks.
- o Finally, eat less high-sugar foods and drinks. We Americans tend to "treat" ourselves to ice cream, doughnuts, and candy way too often. Definitely still indulge. Just limit it to once a week, or once every two weeks, and maybe choose between a margarita and dessert—not both.

The good news (finally!) is that the less sugar and processed foods you eat, the less you will crave them. And you'll have more energy, feel better overall, and your skin will look amazing to boot.

5. Nutritional deficiencies—these can lead to a host of skin problems, some quite severe. I will focus on a less noticeable but more common deficiency, namely a lack of specific essential fatty acids or EFAs ("fatty acid" is used in place of the word oil).

   Omega-3 and omega-6 oils, two EFAs, are truly "essential" because our body does not produce them; therefore, we must include them in our diet. Omega-9 fatty acids–such as oleic acid found in olive oil, canola oil, and sunflower oil–are nonessential because our body can synthesize them from other foods we eat. A lack of EFAs in our systems can lead to dry, cracked, and rough skin. Consuming a balance of the omega-6 and omega-3 oils is essential to maintaining good health. However, our typical American diet tips this balance severely due to an overabundance of omega-6 oils in packaged foods and baked goods, such as canola, corn, cottonseed, sunflower, soy, and safflower oils.

   The benefits of consuming enough omega-3 fatty acids are smoother, plumper skin, lower incidences of inflammatory skin conditions, including acne and rosacea, and a reduction in the signs of aging.

   You can boost your intake of omega-3 fatty acids by eating seafood, such as salmon or sardines, weekly and by including walnuts, ground or soaked chia seeds (soaked as in chia pudding or gel), flaxseed (ground or oil), and spinach as a regular part of your diet. Many people (including myself) take a daily supplement of fish or krill oil to ensure sufficient omega-3 levels. In addition, if you have blemish-prone skin, your body may be lacking in a specific omega-6 essential oil– gamma linolenic acid (GLA). A hemp oil or borage oil supplement may be helpful, or you can supplement with spirulina (blue-green algae) powder to increase your GLA intake.

6. Hormones are chemical messengers sent from glands to a vast number of our biological systems. This relay of hormones works together to facilitate these systems to communicate and regulate their functions. Because our hormones collaborate to make our bodies run smoothly, if one hormone is imbalanced it affects other hormones. What we eat can disturb this hormone balance.

For example, if you have even a small gluten sensitivity, your thyroid gland may be affected. Soy contains phytoestrogens that can mimic estrogen and upset that balance. Sugar and processed foods may increase cortisol, a hormone that can cause inflammation in the skin and increase sebum production. Even licorice is being evaluated as a possible anti-testosterone treatment.[24] While these are just a few examples, much about how specific foods affect hormonal balance is unknown. What *is* accepted as fact is that your diet in general will promote balance or mess with it. Make your glands and hormones happy by eating enough healthy fats including avocados, coconut oil, and omega-3 fatty acids; raw nuts and seeds such as quinoa, almonds, and ground or soaked chia seeds; and green foods including spinach, kale, and broccoli.

Simply Beautiful Skin Nutrition Plan

So, how do we put all this information together to create a simple, yet healthy skin food plan? Let's go back to the pH scale we talked about earlier in the book. We now know our skin is naturally more acidic than alkaline, landing at about a 5.5 on the pH scale. Skincare products should be formulated to test close to this skincare level so as not to disrupt the acid mantle and skin flora (excluding many exfoliation products, which are more acidic). If a product tests at the *alkaline* end of the pH scale, such as regular soap, you run the risk of irritating your skin and causing inflammation.

Conversely, your internal body falls at approximately 7.4 on the pH scale—which is pretty high alkalinity. Therefore, to best design an eating plan that is both good for your skin and your health in general, most of your foods should be alkaline, or at least lean in that direction. **In other words, the higher the number the food is on the pH scale, the better for you.**

If most of what you eat is acid-forming (low pH numbers), your body is constantly working to restore your internal pH balance. With this battle for equilibrium happening inside of you, the worst consequence is inflammation which could lead to skin concerns such as acne, premature aging, dermatitis, and psoriasis, along with health conditions like arthritis and allergies.[25, 26]

To help you meet the goal of eating more alkaline and less acidic foods, I present the *Simply Beautiful Skin* nutrition plan. As you scan the graphics and information below and think to yourself that I must be crazy to call this plan "simple," stay with me! Once you have the basic information, I will show you two different ways to use this plan: one very simple way, and one way that is a bit more in-depth for those wanting a more detailed approach.

PH CHART

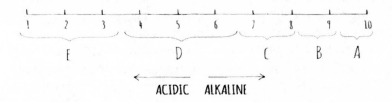

Foods Found in Each Section of the Skin Nutrition pH Chart:

A High Alkaline - Eat and drink as m uch as you l ike, as often as possible:

Alkaline or mineral water, fermented foods, arugula, avocado, barley, broccoli, Brussels sprouts, cabbage, carrots, celery, chia seeds (ground or soaked is best), collard greens, cucumbers, endive, freshly juiced green drinks, garlic, ginger, green beans, herbal teas, kale, leafy greens, lemon, lime, okra, oregano, seaweed, spinach, all sprouted seeds, sprouts, spirulina, stevia, tomatoes, white beans, and zucchini.

B Moderately High Alkaline - Eat in high quantity:

Asparagus, artichokes, basil, beets, bell peppers, bok choy, cantaloupe, cauliflower, chard, chives, eggplant, ginseng, head lettuce, horseradish, leeks, lemongrass, mustard greens, onions, papaya, peas, potatoes with skins, pumpkin, radish, snow peas, spinach, squash, sweet potatoes, yams, fresh coconut, coconut milk, hemp milk, grapefruit, sour cherries, almonds, brazil nuts, flaxseeds, hemp seeds, raw pine nuts, pumpkin seeds, sesame seeds, sunflower seeds, tofu, buckwheat, chickpeas, hummus, quinoa, spelt, sprouted grains, avocado oil, borage oil, coconut oil, evening primrose oil, flaxseed oil, olive oil, and sesame oil.

C Neutral - Don't load up on, but fine to have throughout the week:

Acai berry, apples, apple cider vinegar, apricots, blueberries, cranberries, frozen vegetables, nectarines, oranges, peaches, pears, raspberries, rhubarb, strawberries, watermelon, basmati rice, brown and wild rice, beans (kidney, black, red, navy, and pinto), lentils, oats, soy beans, whole grain baked goods and

---

pasta, potatoes without the skin, walnut oil, hazelnuts, macadamia nuts, pine nuts, walnuts, dark chocolate, eggs, fresh water fish, poultry, and grass-fed beef.

D Moderately High Acid-Forming - Special occasion:

Goat, lamb, pork, salt water fish, shellfish, tuna, veal, hamburgers (not grass-fed), sausages, buttermilk, cheese, canned vegetables, cottage cheese, cream, milk, sour cream, yogurt, ketchup, mayonnaise, mustard, soy sauce, mashed potatoes, cookies, corn and tortilla chips, crackers, doughnuts, muffins, refined white flour bread and pasta, most boxed cereals, white rice, cashews, nuts, peanuts, pistachio, butter, margarine, canola oil, sunflower oil, alcohol, black tea, bottled water (including sparkling), coffee, wine, beer, candy, milk chocolate, ice cream, honey, maple syrup, and mushrooms.

E High Acid-Forming - Never (or as close to never as possible):

Sodas, diet sodas, energy drinks, artificial sweeteners, charred barbeque meat, fried food, fast food, and pickles.

High Sugar - Special Occasion (grouped with the **D** section above):

All dried fruit (including dates, figs, and raisins), bananas, sweet cherries, grapes, kiwi, mango, pineapple, and plums.

Notice there are some very acidic-tasting foods listed in the high alkaline section: lemons, limes, and fermented foods, such as sauerkraut, kimchi, and kombucha. These acidic-tasting items actually help to reduce acidity internally—think of them as turning alkaline once you swallow them. Besides generally increasing your body's alkalinity, ingesting them reduces Advanced Glycation End Products (AGEs).

In addition to the benefits of adding more alkaline foods to improve our skin, I would be remiss not to add another group of foods to the "Special Occasion" section, regardless of their pH value. They are ultra-high sugar fruits. The reason I don't list these fruits by their pH value, but by their sugar content, is because, as discussed earlier, sugar is the biggest nutritional enemy to the skin. Enjoy these foods, but in strict moderation.

We will start by covering the more in-depth skin nutrition plan option. To begin, pull out some blank paper and get ready to complete the work below. Or, if you want the very simple plan (which is coming up), just read through the following information without writing anything down.

First of all, list (or think about) foods you *generally* eat for breakfast, lunch, dinner, and snacks. A tip for coming up with this is to scan your pantry, refrigerator, and freezer and think about carry-out and eating-out foods. No need to list every single thing you eat and how much (although that is perfectly fine if you wish to do so), but make sure to include beverages you consume regularly

Your sheet of paper may look like this:

Breakfast:	Bagels with peanut butter; eggs with ham and cheese; whole-grain cereal with milk; coffee; etc.
Lunch:	Caesar salad with chicken, chicken salad sandwiches on whole-grain bread; leftovers; iced tea with lemon; apple; etc.
Dinner:	Pasta dish with beef and cheese; broccoli or other greens (sometimes with butter); tacos; fish with lemon; roasted chicken; baked potato; etc.
Snacks:	Protein bar; pretzels; tortillas chips with guacamole; ice cream; carrots with hummus; grapes; etc.

Again, the food list does not need to be exact. It probably will contain more food items than this example, but don't spend more than fifteen minutes completing this step.

The next step is to transfer the foods you typically eat to the appropriate sections in a mock-up of the Skin Nutrition pH Chart (plus the high sugar fruits). Using the example above, it should look something like this:

High Alkaline (A):	Romaine lettuce; lemon; broccoli and other greens; tomatoes on tacos; guacamole; carrots; celery in chicken salad; water (mineral)
Moderately High Alkaline (B):	Lettuce on tacos; hummus; onions in chicken salad
Neutral (C):	Eggs; whole grain cereal; milk; chicken; whole-grain bread; apple; fish; baked potato; protein bar
Special Occasion (D):	Bagels; peanut butter; ham; coffee; mayonnaise; tea; pasta; beef; cheese; butter; taco shells; pretzels; tortilla chips; ice cream; margaritas
Never (E):	Nothing
High Sugar Fruits (D):	Grapes

Notice that I wasn't overly specific; I didn't list the Caesar dressing because I wasn't sure where it would go. Also, I placed the protein bar in "neutral" because I read on the label that it is fairly low in sugar (8 grams) and contains whole grains.

Now, I want you to take a deep breath, exhale, and feel no guilt.

This is not an exercise in judging your current diet. If your list looks like our example, many of your food items may end up in special occasion, but you may be surprised at how many are listed as high or moderately high alkaline. We all must start somewhere, and it is best to start with acknowledging our   healthy choices and the not-so-healthy ones.

The next step is to simply scan your personalized food pH and high sugar fruits chart. Are there simple ways to make different food choices that would land higher on the chart? Our chart example person   could decide she will try coconut milk in her cereal instead of cow's milk. She might decide to include her potato skin when she eats a baked potato. She also notices that if she substitutes sunflower seed butter for peanut butter on her bagel, a food item will move up. She also decides to try eating almonds instead of pretzels for a snack. Lastly, she determines she is not married to grapes and will change that fruit snack to an orange, apricot, or a peach. Jot down a handful of beneficial substitutions that   jump out at you. Start with your "Never" food choices first.

If you wish to chart your ideas, it may look something like this:

Never Foods	Special Occasion Foods & High Sugar Foods	Neutral Foods	High Alkalinity Foods (A & B)
		potato ⟶	potato with skin
		milk ⟶	coconut milk
	pretzels ———————⟶		*almonds*
	peanut butter ———————⟶		sunflower seed butter
	grapes ———————⟶		*orange, apricot, or peach*

It is important you always think in the terms of *substitutions* instead of *removing foods*. You never want to feel deprived by limiting what you eat. If you can't think of a food to substitute, then don't change that item. An idea may come to you down the road.

Here comes the simple part: pick only one or two foods to change in your diet at a time. That's all! For example, our chart example person initially chose the above italicized item substitutions: almonds for pretzels, and an orange, apricot, or peach for grapes. Stick with these positive changes until they are a normal part of your life, or in other words, until you aren't thinking about the prior food choice anymore.

Then, when you are totally comfortable with your new diet, pick one or two more items to change. You have permission to stop any changes for a while (especially if you are going through a stressful period in your life), or to go back to your old ways while on vacation or during the holidays. If you need to stop and get hamburgers for dinner one night because you worked overtime, don't think of it as "cheating" on your diet; rather, you simply had to prioritize getting some food in your stomach over a better, yet delayed, food choice. You will be able to make healthier choices the next day.

Also, notice our chart example person initially kept coffee, ham, and ice cream in her diet. If these are important to her, she may keep them forever, possibly just reducing the portions. **The point is not to feel guilty, but to enjoy the satisfaction of making better choices**. I guarantee that once you begin to feel better, have more energy, sleep more soundly, and of course, notice brighter and clearer skin, you will want to make even more healthy food substitutions.

And if one day you are dying for a treat, indulge in some dark chocolate—it's neutral.

Now that you've read through the in-depth plan option above, the very simple plan option is to do everything in your head. What I mean by this is, instead of writing out your general food choices and transferring them to the five pH divisions plus high sugar fruits, scan in your mind your typical food   choices and choose a less healthy one to swap out with a more alkaline choice. Simple as that.

When I started my healthier eating plan (before I understood alkaline and acid-forming foods), I began by eating natural peanut butter instead of the ready-to-eat, sugar-added brand. That was all I changed. I   stuck with that for a while until I figured out another beneficial, yet attainable, substitution. I continue   this approach today, changing up one by one which foods I buy and eat.

And to stay motivated, I always remember that (amazingly!) guacamole is the perfect alkaline food

Tips for The Simply Beautiful Skin Nutrition Plan:

o   Drink lots of alkaline or mineral water. When you wake up in the morning, drink eight to sixteen   ounces of room-temperature or warmed water. Wait thirty minutes before eating or drinking   your coffee or tea. Add a squeeze of lemon or lime to boost the alkalinity. You should aim for half of your weight in ounces of water every day, and you can count herbal tea consumption in   that equation. Personal side note: I experienced a noticeable difference in my skin after I started   drinking my half of my weight (measured in pounds) in ounces of water. I had always thought I   drank enough water each day—about half what I drink now—but those last pesky blemishes   have cleared up with the increase in water intake.

Note: I know healthy alkaline water is hard to come by in many municipal water districts, while   bottled alkaline and mineral water can be expensive. We, as a family, decided it is worth it for us to have glass-bottled mineral water delivered to our house. This water can also be found in large and small bottles in health food stores, or you can purchase a reusable water bottle that converts tap water into alkaline water. Or, you may choose to have an alkaline water system installed in your home. If these options are not available to you, simply drink lots of the water you have. The most important factors are to drink a sufficient amount of water, and substitute water for sugarier and acid-producing drinks.

o When choosing baked goods, rice, or pasta, make sure the first ingredient is a whole or sprouted grain, such as brown rice or sprouted wheat. Quinoa, lentil, and chickpea pastas are also good choices. This includes packaged foods such as jambalaya, dirty rice, and pasta or rice side dishes.

o Eat fruit with the skin. The fiber from the skin will balance out the glycemic sugar rush you will get from the flesh of the fruit. Stay away from fruit juices as much as possible.

o Be aware of the snacks you eat. Plan ahead and have raw nuts (especially almonds and walnuts); hummus or sunflower seed butter with brown rice crackers (or other whole grain crackers) or carrots; chia seed pudding made with coconut or hemp milk; unsweetened vanilla coconut yogurt with a small handful of berries mixed in; seaweed crackers; or lower-sugar fruit on hand.

o Unless you have been diagnosed with rosacea, drink a shot of apple cider vinegar during the day (or mix with a glass of water). Even though it is rated neutral on the pH scale, it will help to reduce the acidity in your body. There are even bottled apple cider vinegar elixirs containing turmeric or other herbs with a sweetener that lessens the vinegary explosion in your mouth.

o   Really pay attention to how much sugar is in your diet. Sugar is snuck into the majority of mainstream commercially packaged foods.

o   Eat fermented foods throughout the week to boost the beneficial bacteria in your intestinal microbiome. If you are not big on the tangy taste of sauerkraut or kimchi, drink a small amount of low sugar kombucha every day. Or you can take a **probiotic supplement; just make sure it is refrigerated and contains at least 25 billion CFUs and 7 strains of beneficial bacteria.**

o   Eat enough healthy fats, such as avocados on your salads, sandwiches, and Mexican food to supply avocado oil. flaxseed oil, which supplies omega-3 EFAs (essential fatty acids) , is good in smoothies or on a salad. Coconut and olive oil are good for cooking. Coconut oil is also great in smoothies, and olive oil is a good substitute for butter on whole-grain bread or as a salad dressing. If you are not getting enough omega-3 EFAs, like the majority of us, take a marine or flaxseed supplement.

o   Try to eat green vegetables with every meal. If you are having eggs or soup, layer spinach or other greens on top. Stuff sandwiches with leafy greens and sprouts. Mix broccoli florets in a   chicken alfredo dish. Replace pasta with vegetable spirals (vegetables cut in the shape of spaghetti pasta). Eat a salad before you have pizza, or, better yet, make a pizza with a cauliflower crust. Layer spinach in your lasagna. Serving a meat and rice or pasta side dish dinner?

Make sure that a green vegetable (or at least some type of vegetable) is also served.

o   Plan your breakfasts well. Traditional American breakfasts typically contain unhealthy choices   such as sugary, refined-flour cereal, sausages and bacon, waffles or pancakes with syrup, and   fruit salad—which *can* be healthy, but is often loaded with a high concentration of those very   high-sugar fruits. For all your meals, but especially breakfast, aim to include a healthy fat,   protein, and greens. Which is a great segue to my last tip:

Simply Beautiful Skin Breakfast Smoothies

There is so much talk about smoothies, and for good reason. It is almost impossible to condense so   much nutrition into a quick and easy meal, unless you drink a smoothie.

Simply Beautiful Skin Breakfast Smoothies start with a base of protein, healthy fats, and leafy greens.   From there, additional items can be added for flavor and to enhance the nutritional value your smoothie. I only focus on *breakfast smoothies* for three reasons:

#1: Breakfast is usually the hardest meal to incorporate greens.

#2: Most people do not have the time in the morning to fix and eat an elaborate meal.

And #3: In addition to being chock-full of skin-healthy foods and spices, a nutritious smoothie is a great   way to start your day.

Ingredients in each smoothie should fall into the low-sugar and neutral to high alkalinity categories of   *The Simply Beautiful Skin* nutrition plan. Start every smoothie with a base of liquid, proteins, healthy   fats, and leafy greens.

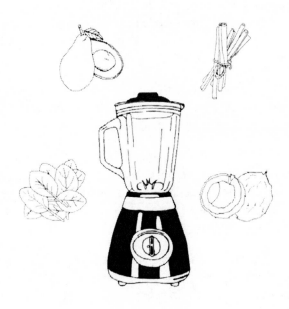

Simply Beautiful Skin Breakfast Smoothie Base:

Begin with about 1 cup of mineral or alkaline water (part of this can be ice if you want a frosty smoothie). Or, for creamier smoothies start with coconut or hemp milk instead of water. See **Creamy Additions,** listed later in the chapter, for more information.

Protein

The skin is made up of protein in the form of collagen, and it therefore needs protein to repair and regenerate. Consuming protein accomplishes this requirement—either in the form of protein-rich foods or from a protein supplement (or a supplement that contains amino acids that will form protein in the body). To complicate things a bit further, collagen can be ingested as a protein supplement; although it won't directly replenish collagen in the skin. It is, however, a protein that highly benefits the skin.

Although protein can be added to your smoothie in many different forms, for skin health nothing beats collagen powder. There are three different types of collagen: I, II, and III.

Type I comprises 90 percent of your skin, nails, ligaments, organs, and bones; therefore, it is the best type to consume. The two most common Type I collagen supplements originate from fish or bovine (cow). Fish collagen has been found to increase collagen in the body better than bovine, yet is more expensive.[27]

In addition, there are two supportive ingredients to look for in your collagen supplement, the first being vitamin C (ascorbic acid). Vitamin C plays a critical role in collagen synthesis and, just like with topical application, consuming it increases collagen production. The second ingredient to look for is hyaluronic acid. Sound familiar? This same component of the skin and skincare ingredient will also increase skin hydration when consumed. In one study, participants who added hyaluronic acid to their diet for four weeks showed significant reductions in skin dryness and wrinkles, as well as improvements to their skin texture.[28]

To sum up, look for a collagen supplement that is Type I, derived from fish, and that includes both vitamin C and hyaluronic acid. Avoid supplements with fillers, sugar, oils, and artificial ingredients.

Other great forms of protein to add to your smoothie are nuts, especially almonds and walnuts. Pea and   hemp protein powder are also good choices. Hemp protein is a complete protein—it includes all ten essential amino acids, which not all protein sources have— and can be added to a smoothie in the form of hemp protein powder or hemp milk.

Protein smoothie measurements:

1 tablespoon (or a serving size) collagen powder with hyaluronic acid and vitamin C; or

A small handful of nuts (almonds and walnuts have high nutritive value beyond just a source of protein);   or

1 tablespoon (or a serving size) of pea or hemp protein.

Healthy Oils

There are two reasons to include healthy oils in your smoothie. The first is, like protein, the addition of   healthy oils make the smoothie a meal—it balances the macro nutrients of carbohydrates, protein, and fat. This balance is important for good nutrition, but also to keep you feeling full until lunch. The second   reason is skin benefits, such as hydration and the vitamins they contain that act as antioxidants.

Avocados are my favorite smoothie ingredient—not only are they a great source of healthy oil, they also   contain vitamins E and B, measure very low on the alkaline scale, and help your liver detoxify, which   helps keep skin clear. And they make smoothies lusciously creamy without the addition of dairy   products. For you purists out there, I know avocados are a fruit, but they contain a great deal of oil;   therefore, they are included in this section.

My other two favorite healthy fat sources are coconut oil and MCT (medium chain triglycerides) oil. Medium chain triglycerides are fatty acids linked to increased energy and improved cognitive function. They also contain lauric acid which has been shown to improve the condition of the digestive tract lining and its microbiome. If you choose to try MCT oil, read the label carefully to ensure it contains lauric acid, as not all brands do.

About 65 percent of virgin coconut oil is medium chain triglycerides plus lauric acid, but not all MCT oil is derived entirely from coconut oil. I look for 100 percent coconut MCT oil because I am assured it will rank high in alkalinity. Another reason to choose MCT oil over coconut oil (besides the purity of medium chain triglycerides contained therein) is because it has no distinct scent or flavor. If you choose to add pure coconut oil, make sure it is not hydrogenated and is labeled "virgin."

To increase your omega-3 fatty acid intake, flaxseed oil is a good choice; plus, it contains vitamin E—just beware, it can have a strong flavor.

<u>Healthy oils smoothie measurements:</u>

1/2 avocado (freeze the other half for another day); or

1 tablespoon coconut oil, MCT oil, or flaxseed oil.

Leafy Greens

Smoothies make eating these super-low alkaline, nutrient and fiber-dense foods at breakfast time easy. And for those not too keen on eating a salad in the morning (like me), you won't even taste the addition of greens in your smoothie.

All greens are highly alkaline, and each has its own specific nutrients.

- Kale, my favorite, is high in vitamins A and C—both powerhouses in helping to delay the signs of aging. It is also rich in vitamin K, which promotes healthy circulation as well as bone and cognitive health, and the minerals calcium, potassium, and iron. In addition, it contains zeaxanthin— remember reading about this antioxidant? It is equally beneficial to ingest it as it is to apply topically to your skin. All types of kale are good additions, some with a stronger flavor than others. I like curly kale and baby kale. Note: the older your kale is, the stronger flavor it will have.
- Spinach is another green high in vitamin A and minerals, such as calcium, iron, and magnesium.
- Collard greens are also a great choice as they are high in beta-carotene (which converts to vitamin A in our bodies), as well as vitamins C and K.
- Swiss chard contains biotin (vitamin B7), a B vitamin often lacking in our diet, which facilitates the work of protein to repair and keep our skin healthy. The skin-healthy vitamins A and C are in there, too.
- A green you may not have thought of using in your smoothie is bok choy. It contains an amazing seventy different antioxidants along with a significant amount of beta-carotene.

Leafy greens smoothie measurements:

1½ to 2 oz (about a handful) of any green, including kale, spinach, collard greens, swiss chard, or bok choy.

Now that you created your smoothie base, it is time to add some flavor and boosters:

Low-Sugar Fruit

Fruit is traditionally included in smoothies to add flavor and additional nutrients.

- Berries (including acai berry) are loaded with antioxidants, vitamin C, and fiber.
- Apples contain phytochemicals that protect against wrinkle-producing AGEs.
- Pears contain a nutrient (a type of flavonoid) that helps moderate blood sugar (red-skinned pears contain two different types of flavonoids, as opposed to other pears that contain just one   type).
- Oranges, grapefruit, and nectarines are all, of course, good sources of vitamin C, but also include   anti-inflammatory and antioxidant nutrients.
- Cantaloupe is high in alkalinity and is one of the highest fruit sources of vitamin A.
- Watermelon hydrates the body as well as supplies vitamin A and lycopene (a carotenoid).
- Papaya is also high in alkalinity and contains beta-carotene and many B vitamins.
- Pumpkin is another fruit option that rates high in alkalinity and is loaded with nutrients, including vitamins A and C, plus many minerals.
- As a bonus, adding a squeeze of lemon or lime will increase the alkaline level of your smoothie.

Low-sugar fruit smoothie measurements:

¾ to 1 cup of low-sugar fruit, or ¼ to ½ cup of pureed fruit (such as pumpkin puree). Larger fruits should be chopped. And while you should never include the seeds of an apple or pear, citrus seeds are fine.

Always include the skin of the fruit unless it is citrus, and (of course) do not include any pits.

It is fine to mix two or three fruits together; however, make sure you don't double or triple the *amount* of fruit which doubles or triples the amount of sugar in your smoothie. It is better to choose a fruit and match it with a vegetable, like the ones listed below.

Other Vegetable Ingredients

Additional vegetables can be added to your smoothie for their nutritional value and to enhance the consistency.

- Cauliflower is high in vitamins C and K, as well as many minerals. For convenience, you can purchase cauliflower "rice," which is cauliflower cut into small pieces resembling rice.
- Zucchini or squash with their skin give you a boost of vitamins A, C, and K.
- Cucumber rates at a very high alkalinity, includes vitamins A and K as well as minerals, and is a wonderful cooling agent in the summer.
- And for a sweeter and highly-flavorful vegetable, try rhubarb (yes, it is a vegetable!) to supply vitamin K, beta-carotene, and the antioxidant zeaxanthin. **Note: only use the rhubarb stalk, as the leaves contain oxalic acid, which may make you sick.**

Vegetable smoothie measurements:

½ a zucchini, cucumber, or squash, chopped 1 ½ oz. rhubarb, chopped

Creamy Additions

Who doesn't crave a milkshake every now and then? Instead of grabbing a high acid-forming milkshake from an ice cream or fast food place (whose milkshakes may not even contain milk), make a smoothie with coconut yogurt, cream, or milk. Unsweetened vanilla coconut yogurt is my favorite because it contains probiotics and is thick enough to make your smoothie extra creamy.

Unsweetened coconut cream is also a good choice. If you want to use coconut milk, the creamiest is packaged in a can (found in the Asian food area of the grocery store); just be aware of the sugar content. Other tasty substitute milks include hemp (also a good source of protein) or flax, but because they are thinner than yogurt or cream, use them as a portion of, or in place of, the water ingredient. I don't suggest rice milk because it contains more sugar than other types of milk. All dairy products from a cow, including milk, can be very troublesome for skin health as well as being acid-forming in the body.

<u>Creamy additions measurements:</u>

¾ to 1 cup of unsweetened or low-sugar (5 grams or less per serving) coconut yogurt (I like vanilla- flavored)

2 tablespoons of coconut cream

1 cup milk substitute (in place of water ingredient)

Spices

Take your smoothie game to the next level with the healing power of spices. Spices customize your smoothie, and many contribute additional health benefits. Look over the spices below and the suggestions for smoothie matches.

- Cinnamon's best attribute, besides its flavor, is that it stabilizes blood sugar.[29] It is known to be comforting, yet noticeably energizing, when added to drinks. Add ¼ to ½ teaspoon to smoothies made with pears or apples.

- Cardamom is one of my favorite calming spices. It has warming properties and facilitates digestion. It is normally found in teas or coffees, but it is delicious added to a creamy and/or a pear smoothie. Mix ¼ teaspoon to your smoothie.
- Ginger is another spice that soothes the stomach and aids in digestion. It is also a super immune system booster. Cut a half-inch of fresh ginger and combine with an apple, cucumber, or orange in your smoothie. Or, see "Soothing Ginger Chamomile Smoothie" recipe listed later in the chapter.
- Mint has a completely different flavor, yet also calms the stomach and eases digestion. Throw in a small bunch of mint to brighten your smoothie. You can go the strictly nutritional route and pair it with cucumber, a pear, and a squeeze of lime (this is very tasty), or lean towards decadence by mixing mint with cacao powder and coconut yogurt.
- Despite its peppery flavor, turmeric is a great smoothie addition due to its strong anti- inflammatory properties— especially helpful if you have a skin condition such as acne or rosacea. If you choose to add this spice, I suggest opening one to two capsules containing both turmeric and piperine (black pepper). Piperine works synergistically with the turmeric to greatly increase absorption.
- Vanilla, as an extract or fresh from the pod, can be added to just about any smoothie for enhanced flavor. I like mixing it with strawberry or orange smoothies. Add ¼ teaspoon, or the contents of one vanilla pod, to your smoothie.
- For yummy, decadent smoothies, try pumpkin or apple pie spice—a slice of pie in a glass! Check out the "Pumpkin Pie Smoothie" or "Apple Pie Smoothie" recipes listed later in the chapter.

Dried Flowers

Flower essences and elements are great to put on your skin *and* in your body. Case in point, many herbal   teas are simply dried flowers, such as chamomile, lavender, and hibiscus, and they have beneficial properties.

- Chamomile is calming to both the body and mind.
- Lavender can aid in digestion and may improve your mood.
- Hibiscus is anti-inflammatory and may boost your immune system.

Of course, you can use any of these on their own or pair them with other flavorful ingredients to add   variety. For example, lavender works well with vanilla or lemon in a creamy smoothie; hibiscus can be   added to a berry or pear smoothie; and check out the "Creamy Spiced Apple Smoothie" or "Soothing   Ginger Chamomile Smoothie" recipes found later in the chapter for examples of how to use chamomile.

Measurements are one tablespoon of chamomile or hibiscus dried flowers, but only ½ to one teaspoon   of lavender, as it is more pungent. These dried flowers can be soaked in water first to bring out more of   the flavor.

Sweeteners

Because one of our goals for a skin-loving smoothie is to keep it low in sugar, it is best to add your own   non-sugar sweetener rather than rely on sweetened protein powders, yogurts, or high-sugar fruits.

Most sugar alternatives are artificial, except for stevia. Stevia comes from an herbal plant and is about   200 times sweeter than sugar. The trick is to find a brand that does not contain fillers (sometimes labeled as a "blend") and is not processed in China, as China does not have the same safety regulations as   other countries. Because sugar content in fruits varies depending on type and amount of ripeness, for the amount of sweetener, I begin with the least amount, taste test, and then add more if necessary. If you use stevia extract, start with a drop or two; if you are using the powder, begin with one pinch. Be careful not to add too much as it can lead to a bitter taste. Stevia extracts also come in flavors, from vanilla cream to English toffee.

Although it may be very tempting to make a very sweet, desert-like smoothie and think of it as your   indulgence for the day, I challenge you to reduce the level of sweetness as much as possible. The reason this is: **the more you reduce the amount of sweet-flavored food you eat, the less you will want it.** This really works! So, if you want to cut your cravings for sweets, give most of your sweet treats the boot.

I do not advocate adding honey, maple syrup, or agave to your smoothie, because your body assimilates them the same way as table sugar. Coconut sugar is a better choice because its absorption is somewhat   slower than table sugar, but it is still an added sugar. I recommend sticking with stevia as a sweetener. If you are sensitive to the taste of stevia, a better choice than added sugar is to include a *small* amount   (two or three chunks) of pineapple or mango to your smoothie.

Smoothie Boosters

Boosters provide additional nutrition and specific properties to your smoothie. Need a pick-me-up? Add   an energy booster. Need to add more roughage in your diet? Add a fiber booster. Plus, some boosters,   like cacao powder, add nutrition *and* flavor.

For an energy lift:

- Caffeinated: Matcha green tea powder provides vitamins, minerals, and a very strong antioxidant, EGCg. It also increases your metabolism; great for those of us trying to lose a few pounds! Add ½ to one teaspoon to each smoothie.
- Non-caffeinated: Black Maca Root Powder is known as a "superfood" because it has so many beneficial properties. It balances hormones, helps build up our immune systems, and includes loads of vitamins and minerals. Start with one tablespoon per smoothie, but you can work up to three tablespoons, if you like. Look for Peruvian Maca.
- Non-caffeinated and sustained energy: Ground or soaked chia seeds won't give you an immediate zing of energy, but an energy that increases throughout the day. The chia seeds need to be ground or soaked (overnight in water or milk alternative, to make a chia seed "gel") or they will move through your digestive system as a fiber source. While this is beneficial, you will gain much more by breaking down the seed's hard exterior. Ground or soaked, they are a great source of omega-3 fatty acids, antioxidants, and vitamins. In addition, chia seeds keep you feeling fuller longer, thus helping with any weight-loss goals.

Other boosters:

- Ground flaxseed provides fiber, omega-3 fatty acids, and antioxidants. Add one tablespoon for each smoothie.
- Ground hemp seed also has fiber and omega-3 fatty acids, as well as protein. Mix in one tablespoon per smoothie.
- Spirulina is blue-green algae, and I consider it to be a "superfood". It is a complete protein (although I don't list it as a protein source, because you would need to add a large amount, which would make your smoothie very strong

flavored), and contains vitamins (including vitamin A), minerals, and antioxidants. In addition, it is believed to increase stamina and improve blemish-prone skin. Add ½ to one teaspoon to each smoothie mixture.

- Other than turning your smoothie into a chocolate shake, cocoa nibs and powder are a great source of antioxidants and minerals. They may also increase your feel-good hormones, serotonin and endorphins (so that is why chocolate is addictive!). You can substitute dark cocoa powder rather than cacao. Add 1 ½ to two tablespoons of powder per smoothie, or if you add cocoa nibs, cut back on the powder.

Smoothie Tips:

o It is best to use a high-powered blender for smoothies, especially if you add frozen fruit or ice.
o All ingredient measurements are approximate.
o Optimal layer order of the ingredients in the blender: first, water or liquid; second, powders, oils, and ground seeds; next, greens; then, if you are adding it, yogurt; and lastly, larger chopped vegetables and fruits and smaller fruits (can be fresh or frozen).
o If you are adding fresh strawberries, no need to cut off the green tops as they add great nutrition.
o Use organic fruits and vegetables whenever possible. If nothing else, eat organic strawberries because the traditional version contains the highest amount of pesticides of any fruit or vegetable, even after washing.
o Refrigerate nuts and seeds after opening.
o **Do not include the seeds of either pears or apples in your smoothie. If the seeds are eaten, amygdalin (a compound found in pits and fruit seeds) may be released, which**

produces cyanide. Our immune system can handle a small amount of cyanide without side effects, but why add the unnecessary burden to our body?

o *Before blending your smoothie, ask yourself the following question: Have I included the three "must-haves"–a healthy fat, a source of protein, and leafy greens?*

Skin-Loving Smoothie Recipes

<u>Berry-Green Smoothie </u>(This is my go-to favorite)

1 cup water

1 tablespoon or serving portion of fish collagen/vitamin C/hyaluronic acid powder or hemp/pea protein powder

1 teaspoon Matcha green tea powder

1 tablespoon ground or soaked chia seeds

1/2 teaspoon spirulina

1 to 2 pinches stevia, or 1 to 5 drops of stevia extract, if needed

Handful of kale

1/2 of an avocado

3/4 to 1 cup of frozen mixed berries

<u>Soothing Ginger Chamomile Smoothie</u>

1 cup water

1 tablespoon or serving portion of fish collagen/vitamin C/hyaluronic acid powder or hemp/pea protein powder

1 tablespoon of dried chamomile flowers (or chamomile tea)

1 to 2 pinches stevia, or 1 to 5 drops of stevia extract

continued

1/2 inch of peeled ginger

Handful of collard greens

1 tablespoon MCT or coconut oil

1 large slice of cantaloupe

1 sliced pear

Squeeze of lemon

Peach-Apple Ambrosia Smoothie

1 cup water

1 to 2 pinches stevia, or 1 to 5 drops of stevia extract, if needed

1 tablespoon dried chamomile flowers (or chamomile tea)

1 ½ to 2 oz. baby bok choy

3 tablespoons almonds

1 pitted peach

1 sliced apple

Creamy Spiced Apple Smoothie

1 cup water

continued

1 tablespoon or serving portion of fish collagen/vitamin C/hyaluronic acid powder or hemp/pea protein powder

1 tablespoon cinnamon

1 pinch stevia, or 1 to 3 drops of stevia extract, if needed

Handful of baby spinach

1 cup unsweetened vanilla coconut yogurt

1/2 of an avocado

1 sliced apple (a pear can be substituted)

Persian Mint Smoothie (Great for hot summer days)

1 cup water

1 tablespoon or serving portion of fish collagen/vitamin C/hyaluronic acid powder or hemp/pea protein   powder

1 to 2 pinches stevia, or 1 to 5 drops of stevia extract, if needed

Handful of swiss chard

1 small bunch of mint

1/2 of an avocado

1 sliced Persian cucumber or any small cucumber

1 chopped pear

1 small lime, juiced

Strawberry-Rhubarb Delight Smoothie

1 cup water

1 scoop of fish collagen/vitamin C/hyaluronic acid powder or hemp/pea protein powder

1 pinch stevia, or 1 to 3 drops of stevia extract, if needed

Handful of kale

1 cup unsweetened vanilla coconut yogurt

1/2 of an avocado

3/4 cup strawberries

1 ½ oz. chopped rhubarb

Note: for a Creamy Blueberry Smoothie, substitute ¾ cup blueberries for the strawberries and rhubarb.

Pumpkin Pie Smoothie (Perfect for autumn)

1/2 cup water

1/2 of a can of pumpkin puree (not pie filling)

1 tablespoon or serving portion of fish collagen/vitamin C/hyaluronic acid powder or hemp/pea protein powder

1/2 teaspoon pumpkin pie spice (cinnamon, nutmeg, ginger, allspice mixture)

1 pinch stevia or 2 to 5 drops of stevia extract, if needed

continued

Handful of kale

1 cup unsweetened vanilla coconut yogurt (use yogurt that contains 5 grams of sugar per serving rather than a lower sugar content yogurt)

1/2 of an avocado

Note: for an Apple Pie Smoothie, substitute 1 to 2 apples and apple pie spice (cinnamon, nutmeg. cardamom, allspice mixture) for the pumpkin puree and the pumpkin pie spice.

Cocoa Supreme Smoothie (for those "I need to have chocolate" days)

1/2 cup of water

1/2 cup of unsweetened coconut yogurt (look for the yogurt that contains 5 grams of sugar per serving rather than a lower-sugar content yogurt)

1 tablespoon or serving portion of fish collagen/vitamin C/hyaluronic acid powder or hemp/pea protein powder

2 pinches stevia, or 2 to 5 drops stevia extract

2 tablespoons cocoa powder

Handful of kale (or other green)

1/2 of an avocado

1/2 cup frozen cauliflower rice

Nutrition for Specific Skin Conditions

If you have skin conditions, you will probably do just about anything to rid yourself of them. Unfortunately, most healthcare and skincare professionals focus only on topical products and don't consider advocating nutritional interventions.

Because of this, there are not many scientific studies correlating food and skin health. Thank goodness there are enough anecdotal stories of alleviating skin conditions by pairing topical treatments with proper nutrition.

Nutritionally, the three areas that are most important if you are experiencing a skin condition, such as acne, rosacea, dermatitis, eczema, and psoriasis, are balancing your hormones, reducing inflammation, and supporting a healthy intestinal microbiome. Eating a high-alkaline diet is the foundation to accomplishing these objectives. However, there are specific food choices you can make to help heal your skin. In addition, there are nutritional practices that will aid in balancing the skin's oil production.

Acne/Blemish-Prone Skin

Unfortunately, there is no simple nutritional path to treat acne. If you have occasional blemish breakouts, eating a healthy diet may do the trick. However, if you suffer from severe papular/pustule or cystic acne, more extensive interventions may be necessary. Add as many of these recommendations as you can while keeping your sanity. If you don't see improvement, or enough improvement, make a commitment to tackle this entire in-depth approach for two weeks to gauge its effectiveness.

o   Balance your gut microbiome by eliminating sugar from your diet and adding fermented foods or a probiotic supplement to your daily routine.

o   Remove all dairy products except hard cheeses, such as parmesan. I have done this, and it is not as hard as it sounds. In the grocery or health food store, look for vegan, non-dairy products in the refrigerated section and on the shelves. I have found cheese, cream cheese, cheese spreads, sour cream, and creamy pasta sauces, such as alfredo. In addition, try my trick of using mayonnaise in place of milk or cream to make delicious non-dairy mashed potatoes and creamy rice side dishes. To make mashed potatoes, mix chicken stock and mayonnaise (I like avocado oil or olive oil mayonnaise) to cooked potatoes. Since I introduced this version, my family has liked this recipe better than traditional mashed potatoes.

Ready for some amazing news? Butter (grass-fed/pasture-raised is best) or Ghee are allowed within this program because of their very low lactose levels and beneficial skin health nutrients, so they can be added to recipes and dishes. (Full disclosure: I do add grass-fed butter to the mashed potato recipe mentioned above.)

Eating out dairy-free can be difficult at first. But I have gotten used to ordering dishes "no cheese", and I truly don't miss it anymore. If giving up all dairy products is too difficult, see if you can forgo regular milk, sour cream, and soft cheeses.

o   Increase your intake of omega-3 fatty acids by eating fish (such as salmon or sardines), ground flaxseeds, flaxseed oil, or ground/soaked chia seeds. Or take a daily supplement.

o   Increase your gamma linolenic acid (GLA) intake with hemp oil, borage oil, or spirulina (blue-green algae in powdered form).

o Eat bone broth to reduce inflammation.
o Be prudent in drinking lots and lots of water (in ounces, half of your body weight measured in   pounds).
o Drink spearmint tea.
o Try the supplement diindolylmethane (DIM), which may help balance your hormones and help   with acne.
o Make sure you are consuming enough minerals, especially zinc.
o As much as possible, stay away from highly acidic foods, such as fried foods, fast food, soft   drinks, and processed snacks.
o Peanuts and peanut butter may also cause problems.
o If you break out on your forehead, it may be a sign of gluten sensitivity. Try eliminating gluten   from your diet and see if your acne improves.
o Sometimes chocolate can cause acne. And when it does, it is usually the cystic variety.

Possible Rosacea

Rosacea is another skin condition without a simple fix, nutritionally speaking. However, on the positive   side, dietary changes will result in a noticeable improvement fairly quickly. This is because specific foods   exacerbate the condition by bringing blood to the surface of the skin; however, other foods reduce   inflammation.

Foods to limit or avoid:

o Spicy foods
o Chocolate
o Coffee and black tea
o Cider
o Soy sauce
o Vinegar
o Salsa or hot sauce

o The following spices: black pepper, curry powder, chili powder, and cayenne pepper
o Red wine, beer, bourbon, gin, vodka, or champagne
o Fermented and dairy foods, which may exacerbate your rosacea

Foods and spices to add to your diet:

o Ginger
o Turmeric
o Bone broth
o Aloe vera gel (drink a shot glass full before bed on an empty stomach)
o Cooling foods, such as cucumber, greens, and watermelon
o And, since fermented foods are contraindicated, take a probiotic supplement.

Dermatitis, Eczema, and Psoriasis

Not a lot is known about the causes of dermatitis, eczema, and psoriasis. Because of this, traditional treatment is focused on superficial treatment of the symptoms. However, we do know that contact dermatitis is caused by an irritant, such as a topical product or plant, and psoriasis is believed to be a reaction caused by an overactive immune system. These conditions need a holistic treatment approach, including soothing topical preparations, stress management, and healthy nutrition. If you suffer greatly from any of these conditions, I suggest seeing a functional medicine or holistic health professional, or a Traditional Chinese Medicine practitioner for additional support.

Besides adhering to a high alkaline diet, the three nutritional goals of balancing your hormones,   lowering inflammation, and maintaining a healthy intestinal microbiome are immensely important for addressing dermatitis, eczema, and psoriasis.

o   Increase probiotic intake. I suggest a supplement in these situations, because fermented foods may cause skin irritation.
o   Consume enough essential fatty acids, such as omega-3, by eating salmon, sardines, ground flaxseeds, flaxseed oil, ground or soaked chia seeds, or by taking a daily supplement.
o   Make sure you have enough healthy oils in your diet, such as from avocados or olive oil.
o   Supplementing with vitamin D3 has been shown to help.
o   Ensure that your diet includes enough zinc.
o   Bone broth will aid in reducing inflammation.
o   Include cooling foods in your diet, such as cucumber, watermelon, greens, and aloe vera gel (a shot glass full–or one ounce–before bed).

Premature Aging Skin

Although we will all see signs of aging on our skin at some point, it is disheartening to see it appear prematurely. This can happen with any skin type, but people with dry skin typically experience wrinkles, sagging, and a rough skin appearance sooner than people with other types of skin. The focus of this condition is on reducing oxidative stress, balancing blood sugar, and lubricating the body.

o   A fish collagen/hyaluronic acid/vitamin C supplement, as described in the *Simply Beautiful Skin* smoothie section, is highly beneficial for counteracting the signs of aging.

o   Ensure that your diet includes enough beneficial oils, including essential fatty acids, such as olive   oil, flaxseed oil, avocados, and omega-3 fatty acids.

o   Hydrate your skin by drinking enough water. Each day, drink half of your body weight (measured   in pounds) in ounces.

o   Eat antioxidant foods such as berries, beans, nuts (not peanuts), and apples.

o   Stay away from free radical producers such as fried foods, charred foods, alcohol, and pesticides   found on non-organic foods. Remember astaxanthin, the antioxidant ingredient found in skincare   products? Taken as a nutritional supplement, it has been shown to balance moisture and improve elasticity and smoothness in the skin.[30]

o   Probiotics will balance your microbiome, which in turn helps cells to flourish and regenerate. In   addition, they may aid in skin hydration and elasticity.

Chapter Seven:
Simple Ways to De-Stress

Perhaps the most universal example of how stress affects our skin is the all-too-common experience of a huge, ugly pimple popping up on our face the day of a big event. I think estheticians work their highest level of magic the day before a wedding, prom, or public speaking event. From these experiences, we understand that stress has a negative effect on our skin.

Stress causes hormones, such as cortisol, to spike and rush through our body, disrupting and causing imbalance in our skin health. **In the case of cortisol, it causes our skin to produce more sebum than it can handle which leads to clogged pores and pimples. Recent studies show that these same stress hormones also cause premature skin aging.**[31]

Stress hormones eat away at our telomeres, the caps of our DNA, causing our DNA strands to fray. When this fraying happens, our cells, including skin cells, cease to function properly, leading to signs of aging—wrinkles, sagging, and age spots. One study showed that women who cared for very ill children had telomeres that were ten years shorter (thus less able to protect the DNA strands) than they should have been.[32] I wish they could have shown before and after pictures of these women's faces, but I can imagine how much older they appeared after their extended period of extreme caretaking.

The good news is that the damage to telomeres can be stopped, and they can be stimulated to regenerate, which will reverse the rate of aging. Pretty amazing, isn't it? And all due to lowering stress levels. Will this mean that if we begin a stress-free lifestyle, we can all have life-long smooth, taut, and   even-tone skin? Not exactly, but reducing stress can definitely slow down the skin aging process.

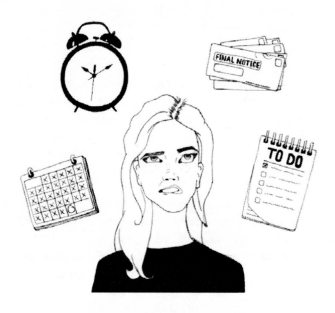

Now the hard part—how can we realistically reduce stress in our hyper-busy lives? Some of the more   widely reported suggestions are getting enough sleep, meditating, finding a type of exercise you enjoy and consistently *doing it,* focusing on optimism, and giving up dieting for making healthy food choices.

One very simple de-stressor I want to share with you is deep breathing. Our response to stress has not   changed since the beginning of human existence. You have probably heard of fight-or-flight (lately   "freeze" has also been added). This reaction to stress is all or nothing, whether we happen upon a tiger in our walking path or our boss nags us daily. Our body reacts the same in both acute and longer, lower-   level stress situations—our heart rate increases, our breathing quickens and shortens, blood rushes to   our extremities and away from our brain (as well as all our other organs), and our body is flooded with   stress hormones.

But, because of the tie that these bodily reactions have to each other and stress, if we change one, we   change them all. Therefore, if we lengthen and deepen our breathing during stressful times, our heart rate will decrease, blood flow will normalize, and the spigot of stress hormones will be switched off. **It is   physiologically impossible to be in the stress response while breathing deeply.**

I understand that if you work in a cauldron of constant stress, it is impossible to breathe deeply throughout your day. However, in a confrontation with said boss, deep breathing will calm you as well as keep that blood flow to your brain so that you can react constructively. The key is to learn to keep the deep breathing up during the entire meeting or encounter. If that is impossible, breathing deeply for a few minutes after a stressful event will rebalance your body's systems and help you move on with your day.

Deep breathing may be why numerous studies of practicing yoga have shown to reduce the physiological signs of stress—increased blood pressure, increased stress hormone levels, and decreased blood flow to the intestines and vital organs. Pranayama, the Sanskrit name for yogic breathing, is an integral part of each yoga class. However, you don't need to join yoga to reap the benefits. **A three- to five-minute deep breathing session at the end of the day is calming and restorative and, as a bonus,   will help you fall asleep.**

Ideas to consider for your deep breathing session:

o   Find a time when the house is at least semi-quiet, and you won't be interrupted, keeping in mind that you will only need a short time to yourself. Right before bedtime is often the best time.

o   Inhale, filling your belly at the lowest portion first, moving up to feeling your sides and back   expand, and finish by filling your lungs. Exhale as slowly as you inhaled.

o   You may find that counting to five while you inhale and exhale helps slow down your breathing.

o   If you are hot or angry, exhale through your mouth instead of your nose. You can also curl your   tongue in an "O" shape as you exhale (a yoga technique).

o   Try to soften your skin and muscles as you exhale. If you are lying down, try visualizing that your   skin is melting off your body (gross, but it works).

o   If it is hard for you to turn off the day as you breathe, you may want to scan your body and relax   each portion as you go. Try this: relax your feet—deep inhale and exhale; relax your lower legs—   deep inhale and exhale; etc. Start with the lower portion of your body and move upward. I tend   to have "monkey-mind" when I'm trying to relax and breathe— this will sound crazy, but when I try to relax "behind my eyes," my whole body and my zooming thoughts release.

o   My favorite breathing technique is to lie on my back and, with each inhale, I think of my body   being very light and lifting, as if helium balloons are attached to my limbs and head. When I   exhale, I think of my body becoming heavy and sinking into the floor, feeling the support of the   ground beneath me.

o   Bonus points: Try to focus on your breathing or your body while you are deep breathing. If your   mind wanders elsewhere, don't worry. Simply return your thoughts to your breath or what is   happening with your body. It is great practice to refocus your mind, as your mind will learn how to quiet itself more automatically in stressful situations.

Or, find a technique that works for you. There is no right or wrong way. The important thing is to make   time to do it—these three to five   minutes   a   day   can   make   a   world   of   difference.

If deep breathing is not your thing, give yourself a gift of taking time out just for yourself—even if it is   only an hour a week (or a month). It may not be the experts' idea of a stress relief activity (or non-activity), but if it works for you, enjoy every moment of it.

Deep breathing, monthly facials, or participating in your choice of a de-stressing activity, such as yoga or   gardening, are specific action steps; but in the "big picture scheme of things", a large chunk of stress can   be removed by *simplifying our lives*. You've already started by, at the very least, reconsidering your path   to healthy and radiant skin, maybe even tackling a bathroom drawer product rehab or substituting some   healthy food choices.

In addition, a simplified and healthy skincare routine can act as a gateway to a simpler and healthier *life*.   Perhaps you will take on the challenge of simplifying your clothes closet, as I did. Or, maybe it will lead to further reflection on all aspects of your life—your work, how you spend your free time (and not feeling   guilty if that time doesn't constitute something "constructive"), and which friends lift you up as opposed   to weighing you down.

I have heard it said that the source of happiness is not searching out events, times, and possessions   that we think will make us happy. The key is to remove as many things as possible that make us unhappy.

In my quest for simplicity, I have begun doing this beyond cleaning my closet. I hate TV ads, so I don't   watch commercial television anymore. I hate traffic, so, as much as possible, I have reduced my routine   travel to a smaller radius around my house (I call this ultra-local shopping). And I hate being confused by   the latest skincare product claims, so I'm enormously happy that my routine has been minimized to only   products I know are the most effective and best to attain my skincare goals. By focusing on this   happiness concept first, I now have a less cluttered mind and more time to concentrate on what brings   me joy.

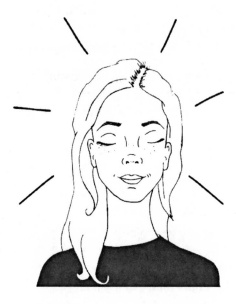

Enjoy streamlining as well as enhancing your skincare. And whether your simplification ends with your   skincare rehab or expands to other aspects of your life, always keep in mind that it is all about prioritizing—keep what you love and what works for you, and ditch the rest!

Join me for more conversation at
www.thesimplybeautifulproject.com.

Chapter Eight: Simply Beautiful Skin Regimes, Skincare Ingredients, and Nutritional Guidelines Tear-Out Sheets

It's here, the chapter you've been waiting for! Whether you tear out the page(s) that relate to your skin type or condition, take a picture, or simply review them in your head, use this information as a guide to selecting your skincare regime. Every person's skin is unique, so I stress that these are generalized recommendations. Please use the knowledge you have gained reading this book, along with your own product experiments, to personalize your routine.

You will notice three regime suggestions for each skin type. Simple A Regimes are for the nearly- minimalists among us. Simple C Regimes are geared towards product junkies; and Simple B Regimes are for those of us who lie somewhere in the middle.

The 10 Commandments of Choosing Quality Skincare Products:

1. **Look for products with a low number of ingredients.**
2. **Scan the ingredient list for ingredients listed in this book.** Remember, these are active ingredients—the stuff that benefits your skin. It is alright if you don't recognize every single ingredient, but you should see identifiable ingredients specific to the claims and type of product.
3. **Scan the top five ingredients for desired active ingredients and the bottom five for the number of preservatives,**

colors, and fragrances. (If the products contain retinol or salicylic acid, these ingredients should be within the top ten listed, depending on concentration.)

4. **In most products, water will be the first ingredient.** If you find aloe at the top of the list, know that the product contains its wonderful properties. However, the product will most certainly cost more.

5. **Glycerin is a fine hydrator and an inexpensive ingredient.** Good to keep in mind if the product you are considering is top dollar.

6. **Remember, the regimes are not set in stone**. The ingredient combination in the products you choose may cause you to change the order of use. For example, I recently reviewed a "brightening" serum that included both antioxidants and retinol. I normally recommend a serum that contains antioxidants for use in the morning because they enhance the protective capabilities of sunscreen; but in this case, the serum would need to be applied at night, since retinol's beneficial effects are deactivated when exposed to sunlight.

7. **Look for multitasking products**. The most common example is a moisturizer that contains a hydrator. For this product, there is no need for a separate hydrating serum unless you have very dry skin. Keep in mind that multitasking products will most likely contain less of each of the active ingredients. This explains why you may need a separate hydrating serum and moisturizer if you are experiencing ultra-dry skin—you will need a more concentrated amount of both a hydrator and an occlusive. Another example of a multiuse product is a cleanser that contains fruit acids in addition to the other ingredients. You may be able to use this as a weekly mask if you leave it on your skin for twenty minutes or so, as well as a daily cleanser.

8. **You don't need to double (or triple) up on the same ingredients in different products unless your skin needs**

multiple applications. For example, a product line may contain an antioxidant   serum with vitamin C, as well as a moisturizer that also contains vitamin C. Unless you would like   to increase the amount of vitamin C applied–for instance, using the serum in the morning and the moisturizer at night–the moisturizer or serum alone is sufficient depending on if you have   drier or oiler skin.

9. **Don't feel pressured to purchase a complete line of skincare products because "they work   better together" or because of some other marketing ploy.** You now have the information you   need to pick and choose the best products for your skin, while limiting your purchases to what   your skin truly needs.

10. **Finally, as I've mentioned, I outline three regimes for each skin type or condition; but as you   learn what your skin needs (and doesn't need), feel free to simplify further!** For example, if you have dry or sensitive skin you may not need to wash your face with cleanser each   morning. You may want to simply dab your face with a toner or skip right to applying a sunscreen.

Simply Beautiful Skin: Dry Skin Skincare Regimes

<u>Simple A Regime</u>

Morning:

1. Cleanser with an oil, cream, or cleanser made specifically for dry skin
2. Hydrating serum with hyaluronic acid
3. Emollient sunscreen of at least SPF 15 (broad spectrum)

Night:

1. Cleanser (may need to use a toner or hydrosol to remove remaining makeup)
2. Hydrating serum
3. Moisturizer, shea butter, or facial oil

<u>Simple B Regime</u>

Morning:

1. Cleanser with an oil, cream, or cleanser made specifically for dry skin
2. Antioxidant serum with vitamins C & E
3. Hydrating serum with hyaluronic acid
4. Moisturizer, shea butter, or facial oil
5. Emollient sunscreen of at least SPF 15 (broad spectrum)

Night:

1. Cleanser (may need to use a toner or hydrosol to remove remaining makeup)
2. Hydrating serum
3. Moisturizer, shea butter, or facial oil mixed with essential oil

<u>Simple C Regime</u>

Morning:

1. Cleanser with an oil, cream, or cleanser made specifically for dry skin
2. Toner made for dry skin, or hydrosol
3. Antioxidant serum with vitamins C & E
4. Hydrating serum with hyaluronic acid
5. Moisturizer, shea butter, or facial oil
6. Eye cream
7. Emollient sunscreen of at least SPF 15 (broad spectrum)

Night:

1. Cleanser
2. Toner or hydrosol
3. Hydrating serum
4. Moisturizer, shea butter, or facial oil mixed with essential oil
5. Eye cream

*All Regimes: optional hydrating and emollient weekly mask or monthly facial.

Ingredients to look for:

Avocado oil • Olive oil • Argan oil • Coconut oil • Shea Butter • Ceramides • Glycerin • Hyaluronic acid • Collagen • Elastin • Lactic acid • Malic acid • Vitamin E • Rose essential oil and hydrosol • Sandalwood essential oil and hydrosol

Dry Skin Nutritional Guidelines:

o Drink plenty of water to hydrate your skin. Ten ounces of warm water first thing in the morning is a wonderful mini-cleanse.

o Make sure you are eating enough healthy fats including essential fatty acids such as omega-3.

Notes:

Simply Beautiful Skin: Oily Skin Skincare Regimes

Simple A Regime

Morning:

1. Mild gel cleanser
2. Light, liquid sunscreen of at least SPF 15 (broad spectrum)

Night:

1. Cleanser
2. Aloe vera gel, hydrating serum that contains oil, or light application of facial oil

Simple B Regime

Morning:

1. Mild gel cleanser
2. Tea tree hydrosol as a toner (geranium and lavender hydrosol can be mixed with tea tree, if preferred)
3. Antioxidant serum that does not contain vitamin E
4. Light, liquid sunscreen of at least SPF 15 (broad spectrum)

Night:

1. Cleanser
2. Tea tree hydrosol as a toner (geranium and lavender hydrosol can be mixed with tea tree, if preferred)
3. Aloe vera gel, hydrating serum that contains oil, or light application of facial oil mixed with tea tree   essential oil

Simple C Regime

Morning:

1. Mild gel cleanser
2. Tea tree hydrosol as a toner (geranium and lavender hydrosol can be mixed with tea tree, if preferred)
3. Antioxidant serum that does not contain vitamin E
4. Eye gel
5. Light, liquid sunscreen of at least SPF 15 (broad spectrum)

Night:

1. Cleanser
2. Tea tree hydrosol as a toner (geranium and lavender hydrosol can be mixed with tea tree, if preferred)
3. Non-moisturizing retinol or salicylic acid treatment
4. Aloe vera gel, hydrating serum that contains oil, or light application of facial oil mixed with tea tree   essential oil
5. Eye gel

*All Regimes: once-a-week mask with clay, moor mud, charcoal, enzymes, AHAs (except lactic acid), salicylic acid,   or a combination.

Ingredients to look for:

All AHAs, except lactic acid ● All enzymes ● Salicylic acid ● Retinol ● Charcoal ● Clays ● Moor mud ● Squalane ● Hazelnut oil ● Grapeseed oil ● Calendula oil ● Jojoba oil ● Tea tree essential oil and hydrosol ● Geranium essential oil and hydrosol ● Lavender essential oil and hydrosol

Oily Skin Nutritional Guidelines:

- o Following a healthy, high alkalinity diet with plenty of water, healthy oils, probiotics, and green vegetables will help balance sebum production. However, no specific foods will lessen oil produced by the skin.

Notes:

Simply Beautiful Skin: Normal or Combination Skin Skincare Regimes

Simple A Regime

Morning:

1. Gel or cream/oil cleanser, depending on whether you lean oily or dry
2. Antioxidant serum
3. Sunscreen of at least SPF 15 (broad spectrum)

Night:

1. Cleanser
2. Hydrating serum
3. Moisturizer or facial oil

Simple B Regime

Morning:

1. Gel or cream/oil cleanser, depending on whether you lean oily or dry
2. Antioxidant serum
3. Sunscreen of at least SPF 15 (broad spectrum)

Night:

1. Cleanser
2. Retinol and/or glycolic acid treatment
3. Hydrating serum
4. Moisturizer or facial oil

<u>Simple C Regime</u>

Morning:

1. Gel or cream/oil cleanser, depending on whether you lean oily or dry
2. Geranium hydrosol as toner
3. Antioxidant serum
4. Eye cream or gel
5. Sunscreen of at least SPF 15 (broad spectrum)

Night:

1. Cleanser
2. Geranium hydrosol as toner
3. Retinol and/or glycolic acid treatment
4. Hydrating serum
5. Moisturizer or facial oil mixed with an essential oil skincare blend
6. Eye cream or gel

*All Regimes: once-a-week mask with AHAs and/or enzymes, or a monthly facial.

Ingredients to look for:

Glycolic acid • Lactic acid • Enzymes • Retinol • All hydrators • Squalane • Hazelnut oil • Rice bran oil • Marula oil • Cranberry seed oil • Emu oil • Jojoba oil • Borage oil • Essential oil skincare blend • Carrot seed oil and hydrosol • Geranium essential oil and hydrosol • Sandalwood essential oil and hydrosol • Palmarosa essential oil and hydrosol • Tea tree hydrosol for oily areas

Normal or Combination Skin Nutritional Guidelines:

- o Following a healthy, high alkalinity diet with healthy oils, and probiotics will help balance the skin.
- o Drink a lot of water. Ten ounces of warm water first thing in the morning is a wonderful mini- cleanse.
- o Aid your hormones by eating enough healthy fats including avocados, coconut oil, and omega-3 fatty acids; raw nuts and seed such as quinoa, almonds, and ground or soaked chia seeds; and green foods including spinach, kale, and broccoli.
- o Considerably limit simple sugar and processed foods intake.

Notes:

Simply Beautiful Skin: Hyperpigmented Skin Skincare Regimes

Simple A Regime

Morning:

1. Gel or cream/oil cleanser, depending on if you lean oily or dry
2. Antioxidant serum
3. Sunscreen of at least SPF 15 (broad spectrum)

Night:

1. Cleanser
2. Brightening or lightening serum
3. Moisturizer or facial oil

Simple B Regime

Morning:

1. Gel or cream/oil cleanser, depending on if you lean oily or dry
2. Antioxidant serum
3. Sunscreen of at least SPF 15 (broad spectrum)

Night:

1. Cleanser
2. Retinol, glycolic acid, azelaic acid, and/or mandelic acid treatment
3. Brightening or lightening serum
4. Moisturizer or facial oil

Simple C Regime

Morning:

1. Gel or cream/oil cleanser, depending on if you lean oily or dry
2. Geranium hydrosol as toner
3. Antioxidant serum
4. Eye cream or gel
5. Sunscreen of at least SPF 15 (broad spectrum)

Night:

1. Cleanser
2. Geranium hydrosol as toner
3. Retinol, glycolic acid, azelaic acid, and/or mandelic acid treatment
4. Brightening or lightening serum
5. Moisturizer or facial oil mixed carrot seed, or skincare blend essential oil
6. Eye cream or gel

*All Regimes: once-a-week mask with AHAs and/or enzymes, or monthly facial or peel. Consider a deeper peel every 6 months.

Ingredients to look for:

All antioxidants • Hydroquinone • Kojic acid • Licorice extract • Gigawhite • Glycolic acid • Mandelic acid • Azelaic acid (or azeloyl glycine) • Retinol • Avocado oil • Carrot seed essential oil

Hyperpigmented Skin Nutritional Guidelines:

- o Following a healthy, high alkalinity diet with plenty of water, healthy oils, probiotics, and green vegetables will help support skin cell turnover.

Notes:

Simply Beautiful Skin: Sensitive Skin Skincare Regimes

Simple A Regime

Morning:

1. Very mild cleanser
2. Antioxidant serum with green tea extract and/or magnesium ascorbyl phosphate (MAP)
3. Sunscreen of at least 15 SPF (broad spectrum) that contains zinc oxide

Night:

1. Cleanser
2. Moisturizer with soothing ingredients, facial oil, or aloe vera gel

Simple B Regime

Morning:

1. Very mild cleanser
2. Antioxidant serum with green tea extract and/or magnesium ascorbyl phosphate (MAP)
3. Sunscreen of at least 15 SPF (broad spectrum) that contains zinc oxide

Night:

1. Cleanser
2. Serum to calm and hydrate sensitive skin
3. Moisturizer with soothing ingredients, facial oil, or aloe vera gel

Simple C Regime

Morning:

1. Very mild cleanser
2. Helichrysum or chamomile hydrosol (or a combo) as toner
3. Antioxidant serum with green tea extract and/or magnesium ascorbyl phosphate (MAP)
4. Eye cream or gel
5. Sunscreen of at least 15 SPF (broad spectrum) that contains zinc oxide

Night:

1. Cleanser
2. Helichrysum or chamomile hydrosol (or a combo) as toner
3. Serum to calm and hydrate sensitive skin
4. Moisturizer with soothing ingredients, facial oil, or aloe vera gel mixed with helichrysum, German chamomile and/or carrot seed essential oil
5. Eye cream or gel

*All Regimes: weekly mask or monthly facial that includes papaya (papain) enzyme, azelaic acid (azeloyl glycine), mandelic acid and/or malic acid.

**Choose products with the least amount of ingredients, and products listed as "fragrance-free".

Ingredients to look for:

Seaweed extract (aldavine) ● Sea whip ● Allantoin ● Chamomile or yarrow (bisabolol) ● All hydrators ● Aloe vera extract or gel ● Vitamin C in the form of magnesium ascorbyl phosphate (MAP) ● Papaya (papain) enzyme ● Azelaic acid (or azeloyl glycine) ● Mandelic acid ● Malic acid ● Calendula oil ● Sea Buckthorn oil ● Rice bran oil ● Evening Primrose oil ● Hemp seed oil ● Jojoba oil ● Shea butter ● Ceramides ● Zinc oxide ● Helichrysum essential oil and hydrosol ● German chamomile essential oil ● Chamomile hydrosol ● Carrot seed essential oil and hydrosol

Sensitive Skin Nutritional Guidelines:

- o It is important if you have sensitive skin to follow a healthy, high alkalinity diet with healthy oils (especially omega-3 fatty acids), probiotics, and green vegetables to help support skin health. This will help your intestinal flora flourish, which will in turn bolster your skin flora or microbiome—something that will strengthen sensitive skin immensely.
- o Drink a lot of water. Ten ounces of warm water first thing in the morning is a wonderful mini- cleanse.
- o Consider consulting a health professional about a food allergy or sensitivity test to rule out foods that may be causing a skin reaction.
- o In addition, eating foods that cool, such as watermelon, cucumber, and avocado, may calm red, sensitive skin. Also, drinking a small amount of aloe gel before bed is another cooling practice.

Notes:

Simply Beautiful Skin: Acne/Blemish-Prone Skin Skincare Regimes

Simple A Regime

Morning:

1. Cleanser that contains salicylic acid (willow bark) or tea tree oil
2. Light, liquid sunscreen of at least SPF 15 (broad spectrum) with zinc oxide

Night:

1. Cleanser
2. Salicylic acid (willow bark) and/or non-moisturizing retinol treatment
3. Light application of facial oil or aloe vera gel

Simple B Regime

Morning:

1. Cleanser that contains salicylic acid (willow bark) or tea tree oil
2. Antioxidant serum that does not contain vitamin E
3. Light, liquid sunscreen of at least SPF 15 (broad spectrum) with zinc oxide

Night:

1. Cleanser
2. Salicylic acid (willow bark) and/or non-moisturizing retinol treatment
3. Aloe vera gel or light application of facial oil mixed with essential oil

Simple C Regime

Morning:

1. Cleanser that contains salicylic acid (willow bark) or tea tree oil
2. Tea tree hydrosol and/or diluted apple cider vinegar as toner
3. Salicylic acid treatment (only if this addition does not make face too dry)
4. Antioxidant serum that does not contain vitamin E
5. Light, liquid sunscreen of at least SPF 15 (broad spectrum) with zinc oxide

Night:

1. Cleanser
2. Tea tree hydrosol and/or diluted apple cider vinegar as toner
3. Salicylic acid (willow bark) and/or non-moisturizing retinol treatment
4. Aloe vera gel or light application of facial oil mixed with essential oil

*All Regimes: weekly mask with charcoal, clay, moor mud, and/or salicylic acid. Add a monthly facial for acne/blemish-prone skin, if you can. If the number and severity of your breakouts doesn't reduce with proper skincare and nutrition, see an esthetician or healthcare provider for additional treatments.

Ingredients to look for:

Salicylic acid (willow bark) • Tea tree essential oil and hydrosol • Charcoal • Clay • Moor mud • Apple cider vinegar • Retinol • Azelaic acid (or azeloyl glycine) • Neem oil • Jojoba oil • Hemp seed oil • Calendula oil • Aloe vera extract or gel • Zinc oxide • Carrot seed essential oil and hydrosol • Sandalwood essential oil and hydrosol • Palmarosa essential oil and hydrosol • Lavender essential oil and hydrosol

Acne/Blemish-Prone Skin Nutritional Guidelines:

- o Reduce sugar intake as much as possible.
- o Remove all dairy products from your diet, except for hard cheeses.
- o Increase omega-3 fatty acids intake.
- o Increase gamma linolenic acid (GLA) intake.
- o Drink lots of water. Ten ounces of warm water first thing in the morning is a wonderful mini- cleanse.
- o Drink spearmint tea.
- o Try the supplement diindolylmethane (DIM).
- o Eat bone broth.
- o Take a probiotic supplement before bedtime.
- o Ensure sufficient intake of minerals, especially zinc.
- o Eliminate peanuts and see if there is improvement.
- o Try eliminating chocolate.
- o Try removing gluten from your diet to see if it makes a difference.

Notes:

Simply Beautiful Skin: Possible Rosacea with Oily Skin and Breakouts Skincare Regimes

<u>Simple A Regime</u>

Morning:

1. Mild, soothing gel cleanser
2. Antioxidant serum with green tea extract and/or magnesium ascorbyl phosphate (MAP)
3. Light, liquid sunscreen of at least 15 SPF (broad spectrum) that contains zinc oxide

Night:

1. Mild, soothing gel cleanser
2. Tea tree essential oil serum, or low-percentage salicylic acid treatment
3. Aloe vera gel, light application of facial oil, or a hydrating serum that contains oil

<u>Simple B Regime</u>

Morning:

1. Mild, soothing gel cleanser
2. Antioxidant serum with green tea extract and/or magnesium ascorbyl phosphate (MAP)
3. Light, liquid sunscreen of at least 15 SPF (broad spectrum) that contains zinc oxide

Night:

1. Mild, soothing gel cleanser
2. Tea tree essential oil serum, or low-percentage salicylic acid treatment
3. Aloe vera gel, a hydrating serum that contains oil, or a light application of facial oil mixed with essential oils

Simple C Regime

Morning:

1. Mild, soothing gel cleanser
2. Tea tree hydrosol (if needed for breakouts) and/or other hydrosols as toner
3. Antioxidant serum with green tea extract and/or magnesium ascorbyl phosphate (MAP)
4. Eye gel
5. Light, liquid sunscreen of at least 15 SPF (broad spectrum) that contains zinc oxide

Night:

1. Mild, soothing gel cleanser
2. Tea tree hydrosol (if needed for breakouts) and/or other hydrosols as toner
3. Tea tree essential oil serum, or low-percentage salicylic acid treatment
4. Aloe vera gel, a hydrating serum that contains oil, or a light application of facial oil mixed with essential oils
5. Eye gel

*All Regimes: weekly mask or monthly facial with papaya (papain) enzyme, mandelic acid and/or azelaic acid.

**Choose products with the least amount of ingredients, and products listed as "fragrance-free".

Ingredients to look for:

Salicylic acid (low-percentage) • Mandelic acid • Papaya (papain) enzyme • Azelaic acid (or azeloyl glycine) • Green tea extract • Vitamin C in the form of magnesium ascorbyl phosphate (MAP) • Allantoin • Jojoba oil • Rice bran oil • Calendula oil • Aloe vera gel • Zinc oxide • Helichyrsum essential oil and hydrosol • German chamomile essential oil • Chamomile hydrosol • Tea tree essential oil and hydrosol • Lavender essential oil and hydrosol

Possible Rosacea with Oily Skin and Breakouts Nutritional Guidelines:

- o Drink a lot of water. Ten ounces of warm water first thing in the morning is a wonderful mini- cleanse.
- o Limit or avoid spicy foods, chocolate, coffee, black tea, cider, soy sauce, vinegar, salsa, hot sauce, black pepper, curry powder, chili powder, cayenne pepper, red wine, beer, bourbon, gin, vodka, champagne, and possibly, fermented and dairy foods.
- o Increase in your diet ginger, turmeric, bone broth, aloe vera gel, a probiotic supplement, and cooling foods, such as cucumber, greens, and watermelon.

Notes:

Simply Beautiful Skin: Possible Rosacea with Dry and Flaky Skin Skincare Regimes

<u>Simple A Regime</u>

Morning:

1. Soothing creamy cleanser
2. Antioxidant serum with green tea extract and/or magnesium ascorbyl phosphate (MAP)
3. Sunscreen with at least SPF 15 (broad spectrum) that contains zinc oxide

Night:

1. Cleanser (may need to use a toner or hydrosol to remove remaining makeup)
2. Hydrating serum with hyaluronic acid
3. Moisturizer with soothing ingredients, shea butter, or facial oil

<u>Simple B Regime</u>

Morning:

1. Soothing creamy cleanser
2. Antioxidant serum with green tea extract and/or magnesium ascorbyl phosphate (MAP)
3. Hydrating serum with hyaluronic acid
4. Moisturizer with soothing ingredients, shea butter, or facial oil mixed with essential oil
5. Broad spectrum sunscreen (at least 15 SPF) containing zinc oxide

Night:

1. Cleanser (may need to use a toner or hydrosol to remove remaining makeup)
2. Hydrating serum with hyaluronic acid
3. Moisturizer with soothing ingredients, shea butter, or facial oil mixed with essential oil

<u>Simple C Regime</u>

Morning:

1. Soothing creamy cleanser
2. Helichrysum, rose and/or chamomile hydrosol as toner
3. Antioxidant serum with green tea extract and/or magnesium ascorbyl phosphate (MAP)
4. Hydrating serum with hyaluronic acid
5. Moisturizer with soothing ingredients, shea butter, or facial oil mixed with essential oil
6. Eye cream
7. Broad spectrum sunscreen (at least 15 SPF) containing zinc oxide

Night:

1. Soothing creamy cleanser
2. Helichrysum, rose and/or chamomile hydrosol as toner
3. Hydrating serum with hyaluronic acid
4. Moisturizer with soothing ingredients, shea butter, or facial oil mixed with essential oil
5. Eye cream

*All Regimes: weekly mask or monthly facial with papaya (papain) enzyme, mandelic acid, azelaic acid, as well as hydrating, soothing, and moisturizing ingredients.

**Choose products with the least amount of ingredients, and products listed as "fragrance-free".

Ingredients to look for:

Mandelic acid • Papaya (papain) enzyme • Azelaic acid (or azeloyl glycine) • Green tea extract • Vitamin C in the form of magnesium ascorbyl phosphate (MAP) • All hydrators • Allantoin • Shea butter • Sea Buckthorn seed oil • Ceramides • Zinc oxide • Helichrysum essential oil and hydrosol • German essential oil • Chamomile hydrosol • Carrot seed essential oil and hydrosol • Rose essential oil and hydrosol • Frankincense essential oil and hydrosol

Possible Rosacea with Dry and Flaky Skin Nutritional Guidelines:

○ Drink plenty of water to hydrate the skin. Ten ounces of warm water first thing in the morning is a wonderful mini-cleanse.

○ Limit or avoid spicy foods, chocolate, coffee, black tea, cider, soy sauce, vinegar, salsa, hot sauce, black pepper, curry powder, chili powder, cayenne pepper, red wine, beer, bourbon, gin, vodka, champagne, and possibly, fermented and dairy foods.

○ Increase in your diet ginger, turmeric, bone broth, aloe vera gel, a probiotic supplement and cooling foods such as cucumber, greens, and watermelon.

○ Make sure you are eating a sufficient amount of healthy oils such as olive oil, flaxseed oil, avocados, and omega-3 fatty acids.

Notes:

Simply Beautiful Skin: Premature Aging Skin Skincare Regimes

<u>Simple A Regime</u>

Morning:

1. Cleanse with gel, cream, or oil cleanser
2. Antioxidant serum with green tea extract, resveratrol, or vitamins C & E
3. Sunscreen with at least SPF 15 (broad spectrum)

Night:

1. Cleanse with gel, cream, or oil cleanser
2. Retinol treatment
3. Moisturizer or facial oil

<u>Simple B Regime</u>

Morning:

1. Cleanse with gel, cream, or oil cleanser
2. Antioxidant serum with green tea extract, resveratrol, or vitamins C & E
3. Sunscreen with at least SPF 15 (broad spectrum)

Night:

1. Cleanse with gel, cream, or oil cleanser
2. Retinol treatment
3. "Anti-aging" or hydrating serum with hyaluronic acid
4. Moisturizer or facial oil

<u>Simple C Regime</u>

Morning:

1. Cleanse with gel, cream, or oil cleanser
2. Rose, geranium, and/or frankincense hydrosol as toner
3. Antioxidant serum with green tea extract, resveratrol, or vitamins C & E
4. Sunscreen with at least SPF 15 (broad spectrum)
5. Eye gel or cream

Night:

1. Cleanse with gel, cream, or oil cleanser
2. Rose, geranium, and/or frankincense hydrosol as toner
3. Retinol treatment
4. "Anti-aging" or hydrating serum with hyaluronic acid
5. Moisturizer or facial oil with rose and/or frankincense essential oil
6. Eye gel or cream

*All Regimes: weekly mask or monthly facial with glycolic acid, lactic acid, and/or mandelic acid.

Ingredients to look for:

All hydrators, but especially hyaluronic acid ● All antioxidants, but especially green tea extract, resveratrol, and vitamins C & E ● Retinol ● Glycolic acid ● Lactic acid ● Mandelic acid ● Argan oil ● Rosehip seed oil ● Cranberry seed oil ● Collagen ● Elastin ● Ceramides ● Peptides (growth factor) ● Plant stem cells ● Geranium essential oil and hydrosol ● Rose essential oil and hydrosol ● Frankincense essential oil and hydrosol

Premature Aging Skin Nutritional Guidelines:

- o Supplement your diet with fish collagen, hyaluronic acid, and vitamin C.
- o Make sure you have a sufficient intake of healthy oils: olive oil, flaxseed oil, avocados, and omega-3 fatty acids.
- o Drink plenty of water and herbal tea. Ten ounces of warm water first thing in the morning is a wonderful mini-cleanse.
- o Increase intake of antioxidant foods: beans, berries, nuts, and apples.
- o Stay away from, as much as possible, fried foods, charred foods, alcohol, and pesticides found on non-organic foods.
- o Take an astaxanthin supplement.
- o Eat probiotic foods such as sauerkraut, kimchi, and kombucha, or take a supplement.

Notes:

Notes

1. *Minimalism: A Documentary About the Important Things.* N.p., n.d. Web. 13 Feb. 2017. https://minimalismfilm.com/.

2. Carver, Courtney. "Project 333." *Be More With Less.* N.p., 2016.   Web   13   Feb.   2017. http://bemorewithless.com/project-333/.

3. Willett, Megan, and Skye Gould. "These 7 Companies Control Almost Every Single Beauty Product You Buy." *Business Insider.* N.p., 18 May 2017. Web. 23 May 2017.

4. Purba, Martalena br, Antigone Kouris-Blazos, Naiyana Wattanapenpaiboon, Widjaja Lukito, Elizabet M. Rothenberg, Bertil C. Steen, and Mark L Wahlqvist. "Skin Wrinkling: Can Food Make a Difference?" *Journal of the American College of Nutrition* 20.1 (2001): 71-80. *PubMed.* Web. 14 Feb.2017.

5. Reynolds, Gretchen. "Younger Skin Through Exercise." *New York Times.* N.p., 16 Apr. 16. Web. 14 Feb. 2017. <https://well.blogs.nytimes.com/2014/04/16/younger-skin-through-exercise/>.

6. Ortiz, Arisa, and Sergei A. Grando. "Smoking and the Skin." *International Journal of Dermatology* 51.3 (2012): 250-62.

7. Grice, Elizabeth A., and Julia A. Segre. "The Skin Microbiome." *Nature reviews. Microbiology* 9.4 (2011): 244–253. *PMC.* Web. 20 Feb. 2017.

8. Michalun, Natalia, and M. Varinia Michalun. *Milady's Skincare and Cosmetic Ingredients Dictionary.* Australia: Delmar, 2015. Print.

9. Michalun, Natalia, and M. Varinia Michalun. *Milady's Skincare and Cosmetic Ingredients Dictionary.* Australia: Delmar, 2015. Print.

10. Tominaga, K., N. Hongo, M. Karato, and E. Yamashita. "Cosmetic benefits of astazanthin on human subjects." *ACTA Biochimica Polonica* 59.2 (2012): 43-47.

11. Baxter, R. A. "Anti-aging properties of resveratrol: review and report of a potent new antioxidant skincare formulation." *Journal of Cosmetic Dermatology.* 2008 Mar;7(1):2-7.

12. Suganuma, Kaoru, Hiroaki Nakajima, Mamitaro Ohtsuki, and Genji Imokawa. "Astaxanthin attenuates the UVA-induced up-regulation of matrix-metalloproteinase-1 and skin fibroblast elastase in human dermal fibroblasts." *Journal of Dermatological Science* 58.2 (2010): 136-42.

13. Borawska MH, Czechowska SK, Markiewicz R, Hayirli A, Olszewska E, Sahin K. "Cell Viability of Normal Human Skin Fibroblast and Fibroblasts Derived from GranulationTissue: Effects of Nutraceuticals." *Journal of Medicinal Food.* 2009 Apr; 12(2):429-34.

14. Linder, Jennifer, MD. "Stem Cell Technology and the Skin." *The Dermatologist* Mar. 2011: n. pag. Web. 1 May 2017.

15. Steinemann, Anne. "Health and Societal Effects from Exposure to Fragranced Consumer Products." *Preventive Medicine Reports* 5 (2017): 45-47. *Science Direct.* Web. 5 Oct. 2017.

16. Nordlund, JJ, PE Grimes, and JP Ortonne. "The Safety of Hydroquinone." *Journal of the European Academy of Dermatology and Venereology* 20.7 (2006): 781-87. Web. 29 Mar. 2017.

17. Bassett, IB, DL Pannowitz, and RS Barnetson. "A Comparative Study of Tea-Tree Oil Versus Benzoylperoxide in the Treatment of Acne." *The Medical Journal of Australia.* 153.8 (1990): 455-58. *PubMed.* Web. 3 Oct. 2017.

18. Szyszkowska, Barbara, Celina Łepecka-Klusek, Katarzyna Kozłowicz, Iwona Jazienicka, and Dorota Krasowska. "The Influence of Selected Ingredients of Dietary Supplements on Skin Conditions." *Advances in Dermatology and Allergology* 3 (2014): 174-81. PMC. Web. 3 Oct. 2017.

19. Reisch, Marc S. "Restrictions on Cosmetic Preservatives Ramp Up." *Chemical & Engineering News* 28 Nov. 2016: 18-20. Print.

20. "What does the sun actually do to the skin?" *That Science Guy.* N.p., 28 Jan. 2011. Web. 16 Mar. 2017.

21. Michalun, Natalia, and M. Varinia Michalun. *Milady's Skincare and Cosmetic Ingredients Dictionary.* Australia: Delmar, 2015. Print.

22. Michalun, Natalia, and M. Varinia Michalun. *Milady's Skincare and Cosmetic Ingredients Dictionary.* Australia: Delmar, 2015. Print.

23. Cates, Trevor. *Clean Skin From Within: The Spa Doctors 2-Week Program to Glowing, Naturally Youthful Skin.* Beverly, MA: Fair Winds, 2017. Print.

24. Pick, Marcelle, OB/GYN, NP. "Hormone Disrupting Foods in Your Kitchen Now." *Women to   Women*. N.p., n.d. Web. 18 May 2017.

25. Jeremy, Anthony H.T., Diana B. Holland, Susan G. Roberts, Kathryn F. Thomson, and William J. Cunliffe. "Inflammatory Events Are Involved in Acne Lesion Initiation." *Journal of Investigative   Dermatology* 121.1 (2003): 20-27. PubMed. Web. 4 Oct. 2017.

26. Lai, Ning-Sheng, Tzung-Yi Tsai, Malcolm Koo, and Ming-Chi Lu. "Association of Rheumatoid Arthritis with Allergic Diseases: A Nationwide Population-Based Cohort Study." *Allergy and   Asthma Proceedings* 36.5 (2015): 99-103. *PubMed*. Web. 4 Oct. 2017.

27. Shiratsuchi, Eri, Megumi Ura, Misako Nakaba, Iori Maeda, and Kouji Okamoto. "Elastin Peptides Prepared from Piscine and Mammalian Elastic Tissues Inhibit Collagen-Induced Platelet Aggregation and Stimulate Migration and Proliferation of Human Skin Bibroblasts." *Journal of Peptide Science* 16.11 (2010): 652-58. *PubMed*. Web. 4 Oct. 2017.

28. Kawada, Chinatsu et al. "Ingested Hyaluronan Moisturizes Dry Skin." *Nutrition Journal* 13 (2014):70. *PMC*. Web. 30 May 2017.

29. Davis, Paul A., and Wallace Yokoyama. "Cinnamon Intake Lowers Fasting Blood Glucose: Meta- Analysis." *Journal of Medicinal Food* 14.9 (2011): 884-89. *PubMed*. Web. 4 Oct. 2017.

30. Tominaga, K., N. Hongo, M. Karato, and E. Yamashita. "Cosmetic Benefits of Astaxanthin on   Human Subjects." *Acta Biochimica Polonica* (2012): 43-47. *Epub*. Web. 21 June 2017.

31. Sandoval, Maria Helena Lesqueves, and Eloisa Leis Ayres. "Skin Aging and Stress." *Stress and Skin Disorders* (2016): 39-45. Web. 9 May 2017.

32. Wolinsky, Howard. "Women and Telomeres." *EMBO reports* 11.3 (2010): 169-72. Web. 9 May 2017.

Index

A

acid mantle, 13–14
acidity, 97, 137, 144
acids
  alpha hydroxy acids (AHAs), 22–23
  alpha lipoic acid, 28
  ascorbic acid, 26, 148
  azelaic acid, 23
  beta hydroxy acids (BHAs), 23–24
  gamma linolenic acid, 33, 133
  glycolic acid, 22, 63, 84
  hyaluronic acid, 28, 148
  kojic acid, 63
  lactic acid, 23
  lauric acid, 99
  malic acid, 22, 200
  mandelic acid, 22
  medium chain triglycerides (MCT), 149–50
  myristic acid, 99
  oleic acid, 99
  palmitic acid, 99
  retinoic acid, 24, 33
  salicylic acid, 23–24, 72–73, 76, 106, 180
  stearic acid, 99
  thioctic acid, 28
acne/blemish-prone skin, 69–76
  case study, 74–76
  DIY Acne/Blemish-Prone Toner, 104
  DIY Oil-Blend Cleanser, 101
  nutritional guidelines for, 166–68, 205
  skincare regimes, tear-out sheet, 203–4

Activated Coconut Charcoal, 73
active ingredients, 5–7, 95, 179
advanced glycation end products (AGEs), 130, 138
AHAs (alpha hydroxy acids), 22–23
alcohols, in skincare products, 29, 44, 45
Aldavine, 67
alkalinity, 97, 102, 134, 138, 143, 150, 152, 153
allantoin extract, 67
aloe extract/aloe vera gel, 36, 87
alpine rose (*Rhododendron ferrugineum*), 42
AM Ticide Coconut, 92
ammonium lauryl (laureth) sulfate, 99
analysis, skin, 123
anti-aging, 82
  ingredients, 15
antibiotics, 72, 78
anti-inflammatories
  azelaic acid, 23
  azulene, 39
  beta hydroxy acids, 23–24
  bisabolol, 67
  calendula oil, 34
  chamomile, 39, 68, 80
  charcoal, 53, 73, 188, 204
  citrus, 23, 152
  emu oil, 29, 35, 192
  frankincense, 39, 80, 81
  German/blue chamomile, 39, 68, 69, 80
  green tea extract, 27
  hemp seed oil, 32, 68
  hibiscus, 156
  lavender, 40

Olea europaea oil (olive oil), 31, 132, 136
olive oil (*Olea europaea oil*), 31, 132, 136
Optiphen/Optiphen Plus, 92
organic skincare ingredients, 18
oxidative damage, 127, 129

P

P. acnes, 14, 24, 70, 71, 72
palmarosa essential oil (*Cymbopogon martini*), 41
papular/pustule acne, 70
parabens, 92
parfum, 45
PDL (Pulsed Dye Laser)treatment, 77
PEG-60 Almond Glycerides, 98
peptides, 42, 83, 86
perfumes/fragrances, 45
Persea gratissima oil (avocado oil), 32
petrolatum/petroleum jelly (petrochemicals), 29
pH chart, 98, 135
pH scale, 97, 134
phenoxyethanol, 92
pigmentation, 61, 111
pineapple enzymes, 24
polyaminopropyl biguanide, 92
Polysorbate, 98
Polysorbate 20, 98
Polysorbate 80, 98
pores, of the skin, 23, 24, 32, 34, 45, 50, 52, 53, 55, 70, 72, 73, 103, 124, 173
potassium sorbate, 92
pregnancy cautions, 13, 39, 61
premature aging skin, 22, 38, 82–87, 108
and smoking, 12
and stress, 173

case study, 84–86
DIY Exfoliating Mask, 115–16
DIY Premature Aging Skin Oil Facial Oil Blend, 109
nutritional guidelines for, 217
skincare regimes, tear-out sheet, 215–16
preservatives, 5, 7, 15, 66, 71, 76, 91, 92, 93, 94, 128, 179
probiotics
and antibiotics, 73
and intestinal health, 72
DIY Probiotic Skin Balancing Mask, 116
for acne/blemish-prone skin, 71
for combination oily and dry skin, 193
for dermatitis, 170
for dry skin, 213
for eczema, 170
for hyperpigmented skin, 197
for normal skin, 193
for oily skin, 189, 209
for premature aging skin, 83
for psoriasis, 170
for rosacea, 77
for sensitive skin, 201
in skincare products, 15
Propionibacterium acne (*P. acnes*), 14, 24, 71, 72
protein, 148–49
psoriasis, 169
DIY Exfoliating mask, 115–16
nutritional guidelines for, 201
Pulsed Dye laser (PDL) treatment, 77
pumpkin enzyme (*Cucurbita pepo*), 25
Pyrus malus (apple), 42

R

reactive skin, 68

CPSIA information can be obtained
at www.ICGtesting.com
Printed in the USA
FFOW03n0349120518
46491560-48446FF